ORAL MEDICINE

Patient Evaluation and Management

Oral Medicine

PATIENT EVALUATION
AND MANAGEMENT

LEVENTE Z. BODAK-GYOVAI, D.M.D., M.Sc.
Assistant Professor, Oral Medicine Department,
School of Dental Medicine,
University of Pennsylvania, Philadelphia, Pennsylvania

AND

JAMES V. MANZIONE, JR., M.D., D.M.D.
Department of Medicine, Beth Israel Hospital,
Harvard Medical School, Boston, Massachusetts

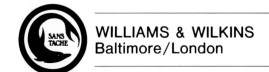

WILLIAMS & WILKINS
Baltimore/London

Copyright ©, 1980
Williams & Wilkins
428 E. Preston Street
Baltimore, Md. 21202, U.S.A.

Made in the United States of America

Library of Congress Cataloging in Publication Data

Bodak-Gyovai, Levente Z.

   Oral medicine.
   Includes bibliographical references and index.
   1. Oral manifestations of general diseases. 2. Dentistry. 3. Medical emergencies.
4. Dental emergencies. I. Manzione, James V., joint author. II. Title.
RK305·B62   617'·522   79-25265
ISBN 0-683-00901-X

Composed and printed at the
Waverly Press, Inc.
Mt. Royal and Guilford Aves.
Baltimore, MD. 21202, U.S.A.

For Judy and Barbara

FOREWORD

It is a privilege to write this foreword to Dr. Bodak's text on *Oral Medicine: Patient Evaluation and Management*.

The author and I and our students worked in the oral diagnosis clinic of a large dental school. Every clinic patient had his blood pressure and pulse determined and a careful medical and drug history taken.

What impressed us both was the large proportion of supposedly "healthy" patients who came to our school clinic for a wide variety of dental services who had varying degrees of compromised health. Many of these patients were entirely unaware of these conditions which might be important to know before dental treatment was initiated.

As a result of our frequent conferences about these patients, Dr. Bodak was urged to write this excellent treatise. It is complete and detailed. The recommendations contained are practical and far from theoretical. They represent experience gained in Budapest, Montreal and Philadelphia. The appropriate evaluation of these patients with "medically compromised health" represents an important phase of the diagnostic procedure for all patients which should precede treatment planning

and treatment in the office. It is extremely important that what we do to, and for, these patients contributes to their health and their life span.

This volume should be a source of ready reference in every dental office both for the recent graduate and especially for the established practitioner. Both will profit from what is currently being taught. The handling of the more common medical entities will be known to the more established practitioners, but it is most important today that the drug history be carefully and properly evaluated in treatment planning.

The phase of dental treatment covered in this book has received major emphasis in the past decade. The practitioner should consider primarily the patient's general health. This includes the possible presence of medically compromised conditions and how these may modify the sequence and kinds of dental treatment that may be tolerated.

This book offers the recent graduate and the established practitioner a logical basis for the dental care of the increasingly large proportion of patients who seek dental services today.

Lester W. Burket, D.D.S., M.D.

PREFACE

This text is addressed to the dental and medical professions. The specific audience is the general dental practitioner, the undergraduate dental student, the dental hygiene student, general dental resident and the postdoctoral dental student. It will also be of particular interest to otolaryngologists as well as general surgeons, internists, nurses, and medical and nursing students.

The purpose of the book is to serve as a practical and useful reference source for collecting relevant diagnostic information and providing proper dental patient management. The following guiding principles are expressed throughout the book: the patient's oral health condition as an integral part of the general health status; success or failure of dental health care as directly or indirectly influenced by the presence or absence of systemic medical problems; dental management of a patient with compromised general health as part of comprehensive patient health care. The procedures outlined are designed to aid in rendering dental service throughout the broad spectrum of conditions ranging from previously diagnosed and compensated problems to unrecognized and therefore uncontrolled disabling circumstances seen in the ambulatory and hospitalized patients.

The book includes a systematic, tabulated assessment of diagnostic characteristics of essential and common systemic conditions, their medical management and their specific dental considerations, such as contemplated drug interactions, preventive measurements, postoperative care and emergency complications.

The book is designed to satisfy high expectations of clinical sensitivity and improved clinical competence, to elicit diagnostic procedures that are of special interest to the dentist, to comprehend the systemic and localized disease entities that can influence dental care acting in accordance with standards of management of medically compromised patients, and to facilitate good cooperation between dental and medical health professionals culminating in the best health care for the dental patient.

Levente Z. Bodak-Gyovai, D.M.D., M.Sc.
James V. Manzione, Jr., M.D., D.M.D.

ACKNOWLEDGMENTS

Dr. Irwin I. Ship deserves our special gratitude for inspiring us to undertake this book and for his encouragement in the early stage of the development of the text.

We truly appreciate the contributions of our friends in the preparation of the book: Dr. Chris Nichols for his candid criticism, many excellent suggestions and valuable conversations concerning the manuscript; Dr. James E. Phillips for the courtesy of his radiographic illustrations; Dr. Herman Segal for his writing on anxiety; Dr. Robert W. Beideman for his suggestions on how to view radiographs; Mrs. Mona Sutnick for advising us to introduce the chapter on nutrition; and Mr. Walther F. Schneider for his help in arranging the text of the Health Questionnaire.

Levente Z. Bodak-Gyovai, D.M.D., M.Sc.
James V. Manzione, Jr., M.D., D.M.D.

Teaching in close association with Dr. L. W. Burket during his last six years of clinical activities resulted in his deep imprint on the material of the book; for this fact I am profoundly grateful to this time-honored scholar.

Levente Z. Bodak-Gyovai, D.M.D., M.Sc.

CONTENTS

CHAPTER ONE
Obtaining the Patient's Health History
Levente Z. Bodak-Gyovai

CHAPTER TWO
Examination Findings
Levente Z. Bodak-Gyovai

CHAPTER THREE
Dental Management of the Diagnosed, Medically
Compromised Patient   *James V. Manzione*

CHAPTER FOUR
Office Emergencies and Statim Medical Complications   *Levente Z. Bodak-Gyovai*

CHAPTER FIVE
Specific Infections the Dentist May Encounter   *Levente Z. Bodak-Gyovai*

CHAPTER SIX
Nutritional Evaluation of the Dental Patient   *Levente Z. Bodak-Gyovai*

Obtaining the Patient's Health History

LEVENTE Z. BODAK-GYOVAI

Introduction

The clinical case record or patient's chart is a permanent file of all the pertinent data obtained. It contains the findings of various examinations, interpretations of the information gathered, treatment provided and complications encountered. It is an official document recording the patient's personal information which cannot be released to anyone by the attending dentist without the expressed permission of the patient. In obtaining, recording and keeping the data, discretion is to be used.

Is is a legal record that can be subpoenaed and used by courts to ascertain the merits of professional responsibility, when questioned.

Providing that a health evaluation was conducted and completed, all the necessary information was collected and no contraindicated therapies were prescribed, the dentist is generally not liable as to the untoward effects that occur during treatment. The most frequent cause of malpractice cases relates to negligence as to record keeping, updating of records and failure to take into account the essential health history findings, diagnoses and treatments.

All significant data are to be recorded in ink: clearly, concisely, thoroughly and accurately. The clinical case record is reviewed and updated at each recall. In general, the clinical case record is composed of the following parts:

Health history.

Examination findings.
Diagnostic probings.
Assessment and diagnostic impressions.
Treatment plan and progress notes.
Discharge summary, recommendations and recall visits.

Health History

The modern dental practice is to interview the patient, permitting no personal or telephone disturbances in the environment where the actual dental service is delivered.

An exchange of communications between the dentist and the patient commences at the first visual contact. There will be no second chance to formulate a first impression. The dentist introduces himself by name and identifies the patient by full name. It is customary to select the patient's first name for further discussion. The ultimate value of health history depends on the dentist-patient relationship, a developing process of interaction between their personalities.

To begin the interview in a positive manner, the dentist should ask the simple question: "Do you have any dental pain or complaint?" Listen carefully to the patient, allow reasonably sufficient time for the patient to describe the signs and symptoms, to express fears and worries. Ask only the necessary questions to clarify the facts. In obtaining the pertinent data the patient deserves professional help if he is unable to find the proper words to explain symptoms, or if he narrates the history revealing signs mixed with symptoms in relatively chronological order. Using simple vocabulary the dialogue is planned to define the clinical manifestations as determined by the type of distress, location, date of onset, mode of development, intensity, extent, radiation, duration, associated change, course, response to treatment, and current status.

An earnest attempt must be made to include all diagnostic possibilities and to avoid unwarranted prejudice by presenting data referrable to only one of the diseases requiring consideration. For example, when the patient complains of pain in the jaw, a diligent effort must be made to obtain additional data that might characterize the disease of various structures relative to that region, including gingivae, teeth, mucosae, maxillary sinus, referred pain from the temporomandibular joint or other sites (myofascial pain-dysfunction syndrome, angina pectoris, hiatal hernia). The patient should outline the area of distress with his finger.

It is essential to include not only all the positive findings of significance, but also the related pertinent negative data. For example, the patient gives a history of rheumatic fever without the presence of organic heart murmur, or presents a history of hepatitis with the absence of hepatitis associated antigen. Since the patient may not be fully aware of a particular disorder that is present and may omit some information that would be of importance, it would be unwise to rely on the interview alone. The dentist should verify essential data presenting patient management considerations by communicating with the patient's physician or appropriate consult.

Generalized, indefinite, answers or vague statements warrant clarification; skillfully oriented questioning should elicit more definite replies. Leading questions that point to an answer are useless, creating inaccurate pictures of the disorder. If the patient digresses from the subject of interest to minimize irrelevant discussions the dentist should guide the discussion, ie., "Tell me more about ... " or "What happened next?" If the patient hesitates, repeating the last sentence, encouraging him to speak will provide sufficient stimulus to continue the history. The patient may not like to communicate an experienced illness or psychiatric disorder due to possible embarrassment. Concern regarding personal matters usually is overcome by the dentist's assurance of strict confidentiality and an understanding attitude. Always anticipate the effect of the question and phrase it in a way not to disturb, irritate or frighten the patient. The manner of the patient's statement is often diagnostic, ie., a depersonalized expression may indicate a psychiatric disorder. It is unwise to point out errors in the patient's use of technical terms. Note the patient's behavior during the interview, including his emotional stability, degree of cooperation, antagonism, expressive reactions, general attitude towards dentistry, anxiety, belligerence, irritability, embarrassment and response to failure or success of previous dental experiences.

The dentist should exhibit empathic interest in the patient's oral and systemic health, explain the known association of the clinical manifestations of systemic and local conditions of various parts of the body to the soft and hard oral tissues. Do not be impatient, do not write down the majority of the interview; maintain eye contact, control your facial expressions, emotional movements, and vocal changes which the patient will notice and interpret. Develop the genuine ability to see the patient's problems from the patient's viewpoint and promote mutual respect conducive to excellent patient rapport. Do not employ nonprofessional, undignified slang. Use an interpreter if a language barrier exists.

Finally, remember, a good history is an essential key to the diagnosis, but a long history is dull.

I. Health Questionnaire (HQ)

In a busy dental office situation, much of the superficial medical/dental information can be collected by the utilization of a HQ. The HQ as a useful, quick overview helps to identify patients having normal or compromised health status; support rendering emergency dental treatment;

and establish the need for eliciting additional details in the patient's complete health history. The HQ can be mailed to the patient at the time of request for an initial appointment or it can be administered to the patient (or parent or guardian) upon arrival on the first visit. Following the completion of the HQ a trained auxiliary person should review the HQ, help the patient understand certain questions and expand upon all the "Yes" answers.

This method saves valuable time for the dentist, but it should be remembered that:

A. A HQ is only the initial step in recording an adequate, complete health history.
B. One must be aware that the patient for some reasons may elect to omit answering some of the questions and regard certain questions as unimportant.
C. Any information, including the HQ or complete health history, obtained by one of the paraprofessional dental auxiliary personnel must be personally reviewed and elaborated upon by the dentist since only he can interpret the content of the data obtained.
D. The HQ serves only as a guide to the dentist in obtaining a complete health history. It raises red flags that the dentist must pay particular attention to when obtaining the patient's medical history. Figure 1.1 represents a sample HQ.

II. Complete Health History (CHHx, Anamnesis)

Using the HQ as a guide, a complete health Hx is obtained by the dentist during his initial interview with the patient. By definition the CHHx is a written record indicating the past and present medical conditions that may or may not influence current or future health services. It constitutes the resumé of the health status of the patient. The rationale for elaborating the CHHx is to consider the scope of a patient's medical problems: ongoing, controlled or cured. Patients with ongoing systemic disorders will develop dental problems and will go to dental offices desiring services. This increases the responsibility of the dentist to select for their patients the appropriate dental treatment plans.

It is the expanded professional obligation of the dentist to obtain all fundamental health information of each dental patient prior to treatment dictated by the following objectives:

To identify individuals having diagnosed medical conditions and health risks.

To suspect, recognize and verify (consult) if signs and symptoms suggest the presence of a systemic disease.

To render the optimal dental treatment in view of all identified health problems.

The additional purpose of the CHHx is to elicit the relationship between oral and systemic conditions; to prevent the possibility of a medical emergency complication; to establish the need for dental treatment in a hospital environment; to take precautionary steps (premedication, chemoprophylaxis) before treatment and to establish the necessary medical/dental cooperation for the welfare of the patient.

The CHHx considers the patient as an individual unit for health care regardless of the specialty involved. It is essential to separate the subjective history data from the objective examination findings and synthesize all the documented results.

Components of the Complete Health History

1. Routine Demographic Data. The complete health history includes the informant, the date, the patient's name, age, sex, address, telephone number, marital status, physician, former dentist, references, occupation, social security number, and dental insurance. The data included here are identification markers of the individual patient.

2. Chief Complaint. The chief complaint consists of presenting signs and symptoms as expressed in the patient's own words. It is recorded in nontechnical language, describing briefly the reason(s) for seeking help. The direct professional answers like "I have maxillary sinusitis or sinus infection" or "advanced periodontal disease" or "class III malocclusion" cannot be accepted without the filter of critical evalu-

DEAR PATIENT: Should you choose to have me handle your dental problems in your best interest at all times, it is necessary for me to have the following data.

Sincerely, Dr. L. Z. Bodak-G.

PLEASE PRINT

				Birth	
Name			Age	Sex M F	Date / /19
last	first	middle			
Address			Zip	MEDICAL ALERT	
Phones: Home	Bus.	Occup.			
Physician's Name		Phys. Phone No.			
Physician's Address					
Name of Dental Insurance		Soc. Sec. No. - -			

WHAT IS THE PURPOSE OF YOUR VISIT? →		General Dental Evaluation	
Hygiene treatment (scale, polish, fluoride)	Root Canal or Extraction	Orthodontics (tooth movement)	
	Crowns/Bridge		
Toothache	Partial/Full Dentures	Periodontal Problems (gums bleed/teeth loose)	
Cavities/Restorations	Special Consultation		

HAVE YOU EVER HAD OR BEEN TREATED FOR THE FOLLOWING?

	Y	N		Y	N
1) Hepatitis, or yellow jaundice, liver disease			12) Seizures, fits, convulsions, epilepsy		
2) Heart attack			13) Emotional problems or "nerves," mental disease		
3) A stroke, any numbness					
4) High blood pressure			14) Radiation or cancer therapy		
5) Heart murmur or abnormal heart sound			15) TB (or lived with TB patient)		
6) Irregular heart beat, heart problem			16) Chronic cough, blood stained sputum		
7) Rheumatic fever or St. Vitus dance			17) Asthma, shortness of breath		
8) Blood transfusion			18) VD, syphilis or "bad blood"		
9) Anemia, thin or low blood			19) Thyroid trouble		
10) Excessive bleeding, hemophilia, nosebleeds			20) Kidney disease, frequent urination		
11) Chest pains over heart or angina			21) Peptic ulcer (stomach or duodenal)		
● ARE YOU IN GOOD HEALTH AT THIS TIME?			22) Diabetes—dry mouth, excessive thirst, hunger, frequent urination		

● When were you last treated by a physician?   Approx. date   /   19   .

For what condition or ailment?

● Have you ever been hospitalized?   Y   N   For what reason:

● Have you had ANY medication (pills, shots or other) of ANY kind in the past six months up to this moment, including allergy pills, contraceptives, vitamins, laxatives, sinus or headache pills, etc.?   Y   N   If yes, please identify the medicine:

● Name ANY disorders (disease, abnormality, lesion, pain, numbness, etc.) you ever had or have at present but are not mentioned above:

● Are there ANY medicines you cannot take because you are allergic to them (e.g., penicillin, dental anesthetic or even an aspirin) because it makes you ill?   Y   N   If yes, please name the medicines:

● Have you ever had allergies or sensitivities to anything, including dental substances?   Y   N   If so, please identify:

● Approx. date of last visit to a dental office: /   /19   .   Reason:

FOR WOMEN ONLY: Are you pregnant?   Y   N   Approx. date of delivery: /   / 19   .

I hereby give consent to the dentist and those under his professional supervision to prescribe and perform whatever dental treatment, dental operation, anesthesia or other dental procedure is deemed necessary or appropriate and mutually agreed upon.

Signature of Patient _____   Date   /   /19   .

( )Patient ( )Father ( )Mother ( )Guardian

Signature of Dentist _____

Remark:

Figure 1.1   A sample health questionnaire.

ation. Select the complaint which is the most significant, the sign or symptom the patient wants most likely treated. Mishandling of the patient starts by not listening carefully to the patient's primary problem and what is the patient's desire as to the relief of the problem.

3. History of Present Illness. Detailed recording and analysis of the history of present illness is the most important part of the complete health history in order to diagnose and evaluate the chief complaint. Within reasonable limits the patient is given the opportunity to talk about the complaint, and is permitted to express emotional feelings and observed reactions relevant to the signs and symptoms of the chief complaint. The historian records an abstract of the character, quality and quantity of the chief complaint as well as a description and definition of the signs and symptoms related to the present illness in a well organized special manner: What? Where? When? Why? Who? Pain, for example, is described by stating the following:

Character (increasing or decreasing, lancinating, pulsating, pressure, dull, annoying, burning, sharp knifelike, crushing like a vise).

Location (localized or diffuse, size of area involved, place of punctum maximum, radiation to other regions or organs).

Time of onset (hour, day, month, year), the cause of its occurrence (precipitating or aggravating factors), the frequency (the last episode), the usual duration (periodic, intermittent, constant).

Severity (interfering with rest or night sleep, eating or drinking, work, exertion or some other important bodily functions, causing tearing or crying out and requiring analgesics).

Association with chills, trembling, temperature changes, sweating, coughing, nausea, vomiting, diarrhea, related psychosomatic status (frustration, depression and anxiety).

Relief produced by alleviating or home care remedies, over-the-counter medications or professional help.

In many cases, the data in the history of present illness are presented in a random chronological order. This is most likely when the patient has several diseases concomitantly or when one disease produces signs and symptoms in various parts of the body in several systems. It is better, however, to deal with each disease or each system chronologically from the time of onset of symptoms. Include each change in symptoms for each chronological period. Diagnostic and treatment data in the past related to the symptoms or signs of the chief complaint are relevant compo-

nents of the history of present illness and these are to be emphasized since they are confirmable. During the period of history of present illness, the historian must never lose sight of the patient's chief complaint.

4. Past Dental History. The past dental history allows the patient to describe previous dental experiences. The patient's opinions and attitudes will provide estimates of prior reactions to dental treatment and indicate the patient's relationship to oral health, hygiene and perception of dental needs. Many times it is worthwhile to contact the former dentist to examine the basis for previous dental care. This description will permit the clinician to develop an accurate overview which can prove to be a valuable diagnostic asset, since it can help to predict the outcome of current contemplated dental therapy; for example, "The patient received three full upper/full lower dentures within a year in various dental offices, but had not worn them judging from the persistence of furrows around the eyes and the facial contours."

5. Past Medical History. The past medical history is composed of well defined, known diagnoses of diseases, the essential positive as well as pertinent negative findings, up to the time of taking the recent history. This information aids the dentist in understanding the patient's overall health status. It includes information about former physical and psychological insults (onset, duration, complications, sequelae and responses to professional management), special susceptibilities (inflammations, allergies, infections, diseases), emotional reactions, and the general physical-psychological makeup of the patient. The past medical history contains the most significant information:

To refer for consultation.

To consider various other diagnostic or therapeutic facilities.

To assure safe and effective dental patient management.

It is well known that there is a broad range of interrelationships and interactions between the systemic and oral manifestations of diseases. Many of the signs and symptoms are present in the oral cavity as well as in other parts of the body, e.g., bleeding disorders and blood dyscrasias. Dental management can alleviate or precipitate, and also aggravate, an existing systemic condition and vice versa, and can lead to a medical/dental emergency indicating that the patient is to receive special attention in order to avoid significant risks of dental treatment. For example, a delicately balanced diabetic can be easily uncontrolled by improper management of the patient for dental surgery, a development which in turn affects the postoperative status in a negative way (i.e., hypoglycemia, bleeding, inflammation). If there is a history of rheumatic fever, one must arrange for special antibiotic chemoprophylaxis prior to dental manipulation that may result in bacteremia and endocarditis.

The past medical history should be obtained keeping the following guidelines in mind.

a. Previously diagnosed significant *diseases of childhood or adulthood: Disorders.* measles, chickenpox, epidemic parotitis, rheumatic fever, heart disease, infective endocarditis, congenital heart disease, myocardial insufficiency (ischemic heart disease, arteriosclerotic heart disease), coronary occlusion (myocardial infarction), cardiac decompensation, hypertensive vascular disease and other cardiovascular disorders, upper respiratory tract infections, frequent episodes of tonsillitis, sore throat, bronchitis, pleurisy, pneumonia, pulmonary asthma, emphysema, tuberculosis, syphilis, gastrointestinal-abdominal problems (peptic ulcer, gastritis, glomerulonephritis, gallbladder disease, pancreatitis, hepatitis), neuro(psychoses), and endocrine system disorders, bleeding disorders (hemophilia), neoplasms, etc., as well as their complications, therapies and sequelae. *Operations and injuries* (accidents—iatrogenic, self-inflicted). *Hospitalizations* (names of institutions in order to obtain the essential details of the illnesses, diagnoses and treatments). *Blood transfusions* and reasons. Previous important and recent *visits to family physicians and specialist consultants* (routine periodic checkups and emergencies).

b. *Medications* taken currently and within the last six months: a dentist must be well informed regarding the basic pharmacology of the drugs that the patient is taking, as well as those he himself prescribes, since problems resulting from harmful effect have been precipitated by drug incompatibilities during dental procedures. The dentist must order the proper drugs during treatment procedures, but he must ensure that the medication is indicated, conveniently and properly regulated or supervised, and all the contemplated drug interactions are avoided. The derivations and doses are critical elements, as are alleged effectiveness and untoward reactions. The dentist should have a working knowledge of the basic pathophysiology of the patient's disease entity, so that these details can be delicately correlated with the pharmacologic effects of the drugs taken. For example, a patient with renal failure and hemodialysis will retain and accumulate certain medications normally excreted in the urine.

Only the correct diagnostic data place the dentist in a position to determine the role played by drug administration in managing the patient's clinical problem. The specific names and doses of drugs taken by the patient can be ascertained by consulting the *Physician's Desk Reference* (PDR), the patient's physician, dentist or pharmacist. There are a great many medications and drug combinations available in the current therapeutic armamentarium. This overwhelming number can be easily reduced by directing the reference reading toward the classes of the drugs, and a prototype representative of the class.

Choose a medication which is most often prescribed for the patients by physicians or dentists. Remember that anything taken into the body that is not food is considered to be medication, including, in certain circumstances, mouth rinses, lozenges and dentifrices. The dentist should also be aware of the pharmacologic effects of certain food substances (coffee—caffeine; tea—theophylline). The patient can self-administer certain medications, including analgesics, tranquilizers, sedatives and hypnotics, or sometimes narcotics. Nicotine intake or the level of alcohol consumption can be abused and the working knowledge of these facts can lead to correct etiologic oral diagnosis and treatment (leukoplakia, B complex deficiency).

Be aware that the "heart pills" may be anticoagulants rather than digitalis alkaloids. Prolonged steroid therapy at sufficient levels can cause suppression or complete shutoff of the adrenal cortical secretory functions and can result in acute adrenal crisis in stress situations. Tetracycline may create vitamin K and B complex deficiencies with related bleeding problems and discoloration of the developing teeth. The phenolphthalein component of a commonly used laxative can be the cause of distressing stomatitis and dermatitis venenata, or erythema multiforme exudativum.

c. *Allergies*: Don't ever miss investigating thoroughly if the patient is allergic to the medication or material you are planning to use. An anaphylactic reaction can lead to death in a very short period of time. Try to verify the presence and identity of the substance of an allergic condition by all the available means (precise history, obtaining older records, requesting recent consults). If the dentist is still not quite certain about the exact name of the medication the patient is allergic to, referral is recommended to either an allergist or allergy clinic to evaluate the presence or absence of the specific allergy or exclude that entire suspected group of medications from the therapeutic regime. The same recommendation holds true for all questionable materials: send a piece of the dental material that you plan to use during the patient's dental therapy to an allergist or allergy clinic, or avoid the use of that material or its components. There are "true allergic reactions" to various substances such as:

Drugs (penicillin, codeine, lidocaine, phenobarbital, etc.).
Food substances (fish products, egg, strawberry, etc.).
Special environmental exposures or occupational allergens (pollens, animal dander, feathers, dust, various metals and chemicals).

The specific nature and clinical course of all prior allergic reactions should be carefully recorded, such as: angioneurotic edema, anaphylactic shock, eczematous dermatitis, stomatitis, serum sickness, hay fever, urticaria, allergic rhinitis, etc. In addition, there are several common, so-called "false allergic reactions," including gastritis, following the intake of acetylsalicylic acid and drowsiness after taking antihis-

tamines. All these complaints must be distinguished from the true allergic reactions.

The absence of hypersensitivity reaction to substances included in the dental therapeutic armamentarium are also noted, e.g., no denture base allergy (stomatitis venenata).

6. Family History. Although the family history appears to have an indirect relationship to the patient's current health condition, it may have a great impact on the relevant diagnoses and treatment plans. The family history:

a. Distinguishes blood relations from the "step" status.
b. Examines the age and general health of the family.
c. Records the causes and ages of death of all members of the immediate family pedigree.
d. Extends to predecessors, siblings, spouse and descendants.

There are various disease conditions which are the so-called "familial diseases," including *endocrine disorders* (i.e., diabetes mellitus), *cardiovascular conditions* (hypertensive vascular disease, cerebrovascular accident, angina pectoris), *renal disease* (nephrolithiasis), *musculoskeletal* problems (rheumatoid arthritis, osteoarthritis), *neuropsychiatric problems* (epilepsy, psychoses, migraine), cancer, allergies and *other hereditary disorders* (bleeding diatheses, osteodentino-amelogenesis imperfecta, cheilopalatoschisis, osteopetrosis, osteochondrodysplasia, hereditary ectodermal dysplasia, immunologic deficiency syndromes, albinism, Wilson's disease, gout and the syndromes: Pierre-Robin's, Ellis-van Creveld, Marfan's, Hurler's, Ehlers-Danlos, Chediak-Higashi, etc. In many cases it is the simplest way to abstract and illustrate the valid information in the form of an actual pedigree (Figure 1.2.)

7. Social History
a. Birthplace and residence(s)
b. Marital status
c. *Socioeconomic status*: Nature and duration of the patient's occupation; essential details of environmental influences such as toxic agents, dust, temperature, illumination, ventilation (these questions are significant in the diagnosis of "occupational" diseases);

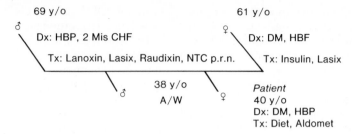

Figure 1.2 Family pedigree. Dx = diagnosis; Tx = treatment; HBP = high blood pressure; MI = myocardial infarction; CHF = congestive heart failure; DM = diabetes mellitus.

education level, the monthly or yearly income.

d. Hobbies, habits, addictions (nature, duration, amount, frequency): alcohol (ETOH), coffee intake; tobacco (smoking, chewing); drug abuse (prescribed or not, "street drug," over-the-counter medication); Food, fluid consumption (hot-spicy, temperature).

8. Review of Systems. The information in this part expands upon disorders and problems of the constitution, head, eyes, ears, nose and throat, skin, appendages, bone, joints and muscles, heart and vascular system, lungs, air passages, gastrointestinal tract, genitourinary system, blood and blood forming tissues, endocrine organs and neurologic functions, oral and paraoral structures. The review of systems is essentially a systematic questioning and recording of the signs and symptoms of disease processes applied to organ systems.

The patient often does not remember all the experienced diseases; therefore, remind the patient by covering the clinical manifestations of the major systemic diseases. A patient can be:

Ignorant of abnormal functions.

Unaccustomed to some specific normal physiologic activity.

Adapted slowly to significantly compromised functions. All these points are revealed by the systemic inventory of the various systems of the body. The dentist should include all the significant illnesses in order to protect himself and his patient from health hazards during the dental therapy.

It is not within the scope of duties of the dentist to establish clinical diagnosis of systemic diseases; however, the contemporary dental practitioner is expected to suspect, recognize, record and consult in such questions. A useful and simple method to refresh the patient's memory-recall is to list the essential signs and symptoms of diseases related to different systems of the body proper.

a. *Constitution*: A picture of the patient's well being, the overall health image of the patient. History of generalized fatigue, weakness, prostration, listlessness, irritability, emotional instability, developmental state, nutritional condition, loss of appetite (anorexia); significant weight gain (obesity); or loss of weight (cachexia); sleepiness (somnolence); inability to sleep (insomnia); low grade fever (chronic infection, tuberculosis, cancer); frequent chills, severe fever, sweats, condition of pregnancy; thirst (uncontrolled diabetes mellitus, diabetes insipidus, dehydration), polyphagia; cold intolerance (hypothyroidism, adult hypopituitarism), heat intolerance (hyperthyroidism).

b. *Head, eyes, ears, nose and throat*
(1) Head

Headache: diffuse, unrelated to any nerve distribution, or confined to one side or to a region of the head (occipital, temporal, frontal), time of occurrence, frequency, character of the pain, associated disorder such as hypotension, hypertension, glomerulonephritis, anemia, diabetes mellitus, hepatitis, pyelonephritis, febrile and toxic states; sepsis (dental focus, tonsils, paranasal air sinuses), deviated nasal septum, nasal congestion, glaucoma, defective vision, otitis, hearing deficit, constipation, indigestion, polluted air, overwork, tension, worry, anxiety; organic brain disease (neoplasm, aneurysm, hydrocephalus, encephalitis), meningitis; sick headache (migraine), muscle tension headache.

Dizziness (vertigo, giddiness): disturbed equilibrium as seen in Meniere's disease, inner ear problems; toxic state (food poisoning, ETOH, salicylism), hypertension, organic brain lesion, epilepsy. Note any associated nausea and vomiting or neurologic symptoms or signs.

Facial expression: voluntary or involuntary muscle movements.

Disordered sensation (hyperesthesia, paresthesia, anesthesia).

(2) Eyes

Ophthalmodynia (pain); *lacrimation* (foreign body in the eye, conjunctivitis, red eyes in chronic renal failure, acute glaucoma); *eyestrain* (asthenopia); *eyeglasses* (myopia, hypermetropia); visual disturbances including hemeralopia, daltonism; *diplopia* (double vision); cataracts, visual field defects, transient loss of vision (amaurosis fugax); photophobia, hordeolosis, visual hallucinations; *ophthalmoplegia* (diabetes mellitus and Horner's syndrome); strabismus; *exophthalmos or proptosis* (hyperthyroidism).

(3) Ears

Pain; *tinnitus* (ringing or buzzing sensations); and complete or partial loss of auditory perception as related to *conduction problems* (cerumen, foreign body); injuries or *infections of various parts of the ear* (otitis); otosclerosis, Meniere's disease; *systemic influences* (anemia, hypothyroidism, endemic cretinism, hypertension); disturbances of the *central nervous system* (psychic disorders, cerebral edema and hyperemia, nervous tension, cortical and organic cerebral lesions, disease states of acoustic and cochlear nerves); mastoiditis, auditory hallucinations.

(4) Nose

Nasal discharge (rhinorrhea related to allergy, common cold, coryza syphilitica); *epistaxis* (blood dyscrasia, cancer, trauma caused by "nose picking," foreign body, erythema multiforme exudativum, hereditary hemorrhagic telangiectasia); olfactory hallucinations; *hyperosmia, anosmia* (rhinitis, olfactory neuritis, gumma, neurasthenia, psychic disorders); nasopharyngitis; nasosinusitis; *obstruction* (congestion, foreign body, adenoid problems, neoplasm).

(5) Throat

Pain, dysphagia, irritation, dryness, cough, postnasal secretion are manifestations of pharyngitis; *hoarseness,* (hyper-parathyroidism); pain; *dysphonia, aphonia* (atonic vocal cords, inflammation of recurrent laryngeal nerve); tickling sensation and cough are present in laryngitis, tumor; spasmodic cough, expiratory and inspiratory dyspnea of laryngospasm and impeding laryngeal occlusion, asphyxia; *tonsillitis* (pain on deglutition, "sore throat"), *laryngeal stridor* (tetany).

c. *Skin and appendages. Pruritus* (mycotic infections, chronic renal failure, secondary hyperparathyroidism, glomerulonephritis, hepatitis, malignant lymphoma, intestinal parasites); *moist* (increased perspiration due to hot beverages and high environmental temperature, excessive physical exercise, emotional stress, pulmonary tuberculosis, septic fever, neuralgias, migraine, hyperthyroidism); *cold* (stress, fear, depression); *hot-flushed, hyperemic* (pyrexia, infection and inflammation, Cushing's syndrome, alcoholism, emotional overexcitement, actinic dermatitis); *dry* (hypoparathyroidism, hypothyroidism, nutritional deficiency); *scaling* (eczematous or seborrheic dermatitis, lupus erythematosus, psoriasis, tinea); *easy bruising and purpuric extravasations, purplish striae* (Cushing's syndrome, blood dyscrasias, rheumatism, debility, senility); *pallor* (occult bleeding and anemia, severe acute hemorrhage, vasovagal syncope, faintness, cachexia due to advanced malignant disease, undernutrition, renal disease, 3° syphilis, tuberculosis, leukemia); *yellow* (hepatitis viral, chemical or other type, pernicious anemia, biliary problems); *cyanotic-purplish* (circulatory or respiratory insufficiency, or decompensation, polycythemia); *sores, exanthems, ulceration, pigmentation changes* (Addison's disease, Albright's and Jaffe's syndrome, chronic renal failure, melanoma, Peutz-Jeghers syndrome, and indolent superficial and superinfected cutaneous ulcers in Cushing's syndrome, hypoparathyroidism, diabetes mellitus, tabes dorsalis); *hives* (hypersensitivity); *edema* (cardiac, and renal decompensation); the date, type, reason and result (positive, negative, degree) of *skin tests,* such as PPD or tine for tuberculosis, Kveim, allergic reaction in stomatitis or dermatitis venenata/medicamentosa; *cutaneous sensory changes* (diabetes mellitus, megaloblastic anemia, neurolues, chronic alcoholism, multiple sclerosis);

hemochromatosis (iron overloading, porphyria, diabetes mellitus, nephropathy); *loss or changes in usual hair distribution, alopecia* (syphilis, hereditary ectodermal dysplasia, hypoparathyroidism); *sparse hair and thin eyebrows in hypothyroidism; thick hairy skin in acromegaly; loss of pubic, axillary, etc., hair* in adult hypopituitarism; *hirsutism* in Cushing's syndrome. *Nail changes—koilonychia or spoon-shaped* (anemia); *extensive curvature* (chronic circulatory or pulmonary disorder, pachyperiostosis); *deformity and atrophy* (hyperthyroidism, hypoparathyroidism, status post-traumaticus, onychomycosis); *splitting or onychorrhexis* (brittle nails) and *longitudinal striations* (vitamin deficiency, dental and intestinal focal infections); *dark blue due to subungual hematoma* (trauma, bleeding disorder); *rhythmic blanching* (anemia, wide pulse pressure, aortic insufficiency); *split subungual hemorrhages* in subacute bacterial endocarditis; *cyanotic* or *clubbed* (respiratory or circulatory decompensation).

d. *Bones, joints and muscles: Pathologic and traumatic bone fractures* (osteogenesis imperfecta, osteoporosis, hyperparathyroidism, Cushing's syndrome, Maroteaux-Lamy syndrome, Paget's disease of bone, fibrous dysplasia of bone, Albers-Schönberg disease); *malformations and deformities* (vitamin D deficiency, familial hypophosphatemia, thalassemia major, hypothyroidism, acromegaly, hypophosphatasemia, various bone tumors, chronic renal failure, osteomalacia, and disotoses, like cleidocranial, craniofacial, mandibulofacial, chondrodystrophia fatalis); *retarded skeletal growth* (childhood hypopituitarism, endemic cretinism); *increased growth* (gigantism—large head, hands, feet, teeth; acromegaly—broad hands, fingers, nose, thorax, thick lips, bow legs, "rolling gait," prognathism, coarse facial features); *bone pain* (various bone infections, fibrous dysplasia of bone, bleeding disorders and blood dyscrasias, hyperparathyroidism with osteitis fibrosa cystica); *joint stiffness and limitations of movements, pain* (specific infections; osteoarthritis or degenerative joint disease; attacks of gout in chronic leukemia, gout per se; rheumatoid arthritis; fibrous ankylosis; hyperparathyroidism; prolonged immobilization; chondrodystrophia fetalis); *joint laxity and hyperextensibility* (Down's syndrome, osteogenesis imperfecta, Marfan-Archard syndrome, Ehlers-Danlos syndrome); *joint crepitation* (chronic sustained trauma, abnormal joint surface); *myalgia* (muscle pain due to nonspecific inflammation or myositis, trauma); *rapidly developing muscle weakness during activities such as speech, facial expression, mastication and deglutition* (dysphagia); *ptosis of the eyelids* (myotonias, myasthenia gravis); *painful, prolonged irregular spasmodic muscle contractions* (myotonia); *inability to run, waddling gait* (chronic renal failure); *unable to close the eyes, to smile,* to whistle (muscular dystrophy); *muscle fasciculations* (hyperparathyroidism); *muscle wasting* (atrophy due to nutritional disturbances, cachexia, chronic renal failure, disuse, aging); *enlargement* (macroglossia, masseter hypertrophy); *tremor* (Parkinson's disease, chronic alcoholism, hyperthyroidism, senility, excitement, excessive physical exertion, encephalopathy); *paralysis* (spastic due to upper motor neuron disease, flaccid as seen in lower motor neuron lesion, Parkinson's disease, chronic alcoholism, localized in Bell's palsy); *muscle cramps, twitching, claudication* (chronic renal failure, atheroscelortic cardiovascular disease, diabetes mellitus, glomerulonephritis); *seizures, tetanic convulsions, muscle spasms, cramps, "carpopedal spasms"* (acute renal failure, primary aldosteronism, hypoparathyroidism, electrolyte abnormalities).

e. *Cardiovascular (CV):* Table 1.1 lists all the major cardiovascular disorders and the related signs and symptoms.

(1) Episodes of labored, wheezing respiration (cardiac asthma).

(2) Blood tinged frothy expectoration.

(3) Dull, deep, visceral, boring, gripping discomfort, pain sensation (cardiodynia) in the substernal area, or radiating pain in the left shoulder, arm, back, neck and mandible.

(4) Syncope upon suddenly assuming the upright posture (orthostatic hypotension), and upon physical exercise.

(5) Peripheral dependent edema, governed by gravity, e.g., feet, ankles, sacral region.

Table 1.1
Cardiovascular Disorders

Symptom	Congenital heart disease	Left ventricular failure	Right ventricular failure	Mitral stenosis	Mitral insufficiency	Aortic stenosis	Aortic insufficiency	Idiopathic hypertrophic subaortic stenosis	Pulmonary embolism, infarction, pneumonia	Primary pulmonary hypertension	Arterial hypertension	Angina pectoris	Acute myocardial infarction	Hypotensive states	Thrombophlebitis, phlebothrombosis
Dyspnea on exertion	+	+	+	+	+	+	+	+	+	+	+	+			
Orthopnea (recumbent dyspnea)		+		+	+	+	+	+			+		+		
Dusky cyanosis	+	+	+										+		
Paroxysmal nocturnal dyspnea (1)		+		+	+	+	+	+	+	+	+				
Hemoptysis (2)		+		+					+						
Fever									+				+		+
Angina pectoris (3)	+	+	+	+	+	+	+	+	+	+	+	+	+		
Crushing, intense, prolonged substernal or radiating pain		+	+	+		+	+				+	+	+		
Clubbing of the fingers, toes	+	+	+			+				+					
Effort syncope (4)	+					+	+	+		+			+	+	
Fatigue, weakness		+	+	+	+	+			+	+	+		+		
Night coughing		+		+	+				+		+		+		
Peripheral edema (5)			+	+	+					+			+		+
Hepatomegaly (6)			+	+	+					+			+		
Distended cervical veins			+	+					+	+					
Nail cyanosis	+	+	+												
Mottled cyanosis															+
Splenomegaly (6)			+	+	+					+					
Increased nocturnal frequency		+	+							+	+				
Anorexia		+	+							+					
Cardiac cachexia	+		+			+				+					
Headache			+							+	+				
Insomnia															
Restlessness, anxiety, irritability (neurasthenia)			+							+	+		+	+	
Oliguria		+	+											+	
Nocturnal angina (7)		+						+			+	+	+		
Cheyne-Stokes respiration (8)		+						+					+		

Table 1.1—Continued

	Congenital heart disease	Left ventricular failure	Right ventricular failure	Mitral stenosis	Mitral insufficiency	Aortic stenosis	Aortic insufficiency	Idiopathic hypertrophic subaortic stenosis	Pulmonary embolism infarction, pneumonia	Primary pulmonary hypertension	Arterial hypertension	Angina pectoris	Acute myocardial infarction	Hypotensive states	Thrombophlebitis, phlebothrombosis
Cold sweating		+										+	+	+	
Common fainting (vasovagal syncope)			+			+				+			+	+	
Local pain, edema (9)															+
Blurred vision, scotomas											+				
Intermittent claudication											+				
Epistaxis											+				

(6) Systemic venous congestion and generalized edema (anasarca).

(7) Precordial distress in supine position.

(8) Periodic breathing: alternate periods of apnea and hyperventilation.

(9) Local pain, tenderness over the involved area, and unexplained increase of the circumference of the extremity.

f. *Respiratory:* Persistent productive *cough* and *sputum production, fatigue, general prostration, anorexia, wasting, chest pain* (pulmonary carcinoma, chronic pulmonary tuberculosis, pneumonia, chronic bronchitis, bronchiectasis); *night sweats* (chronic pulmonary tuberculosis); *hemoptysis* (pulmonary edema, pneumonia, pulmonary carcinoma, chronic pulmonary tuberculosis, bronchitis); *clubbing of the fingers* (pulmonary carcinoma, bronchiectasis, chronic obstructive pulmonary disease); *cyanotic lips, mucous membranes, and nail beds* (pneumonia, pulmonary edema chronic obstructive pulmonary disease, bronchiectasis); *paroxysmal nocturnal dyspnea, orthopnea* (pulmonary edema); *cough with wheezing and sensation of chest tightness* (asthma); *dyspnea* (bronchiectasis, asthma, emphysema, pulmonary edema, pulmonary carcinoma); chest pain in tuberculosis of the pleura; *chills and fever* (chronic pulmonary tuberculosis, tuberculosis of the pleura, pleuritis, pulmonary embolism, pneumonia); *chest x-rays* (dates, reasons, results).

g. *Gastrointestinal (GI): Difficult swallowing or dysphagia is present in Plummer-Vinson syndrome; cranial nerve lesion* (V, VII, IX, X, XI); *and motor dysfunction of the muscles of the tongue, pharynx, upper third of the esophagus; motor neuron disturbance* (systemic lupus erythematosus, scleroderma, achalasia, multiple sclerosis, Parkinsonism, alcoholic neuropathy, bulbar palsy); *emotional upset and anxiety related "lump in the throat"* (globus hystericus); *xerostomia* (Sjögren's syndrome, uncontrolled diabetes, chronic renal failure, nicotine toxication); *sialorrhea* (peptic ulcer, Zollinger-Ellison syndrome); *gagging and regurgitation of the food, liquid through the nasal cavity* (stenotic lumen, mechanical obstruction, eg., progressive systemic sclerosis, carcinoma); *glossitis, angular cheilosis* (megaloblastic

Table 1.2
Hematopoietic Disorders

	Megaloblastic anemia	Acute hemolytic anemia	Aplastic anemia	Iron deficiency anemia	Hemolytic anemia	Sickle cell anemia	Thalassemia major	Methemoglobinemia	Polycythemia	Agranulocytosis, leukopenia	Acute leukemia	Chronic leukemia	Lymphomas	Thrombocytopenic purpura	Classic hemophilia	Vascular hemophilia
Pallor	+		+	+	+		+			+	+					
Icterus		+			+	+	+									
Dusky red cyanotic plethora								+	+							
Bruising, hemorrhages (1)	+		+								+	+	+	+	+	+
Nerve lesions (2)	+												+	+	+	+
Tachycardia	+	+	+	+	+			+	+							
Orthostatic hypotension, syncope		+		+	+			+	+							
Palpitation	+	+		+				+	+							
Dyspnea	+	+	+	+	+			+	+							
Asthenia (3)	+	+	+	+				+	+	+	+	+	+			
Anorexia, weight loss	+			+							+	+	+			
Headache		+		+				+	+	+	+					
Tinnitus, dizziness				+				+	+		+					
Dysphagia				+						+						
Lymphadenopathy	+	+			+	+					+	+	+			
Infections										+	+	+	+			
Pruritus, night sweats												+	+			
Argyll Robertson pupil	+															

Table 1.3
Endocrine Disorders

	Adult hypopituitarism	Adult hyperpituitarism (acromegaly)	Diabetes insipidus	Hyperthyroidism and Graves' disease	Thyroiditis	Hypothyroidism and myxedema	Endemic goiter	Endemic cretinism	Addison's disease	Cushing's syndrome	Primary aldosteronism	Hyperparathyroidism	Hypoparathyroidism	Diabetes mellitus (juvenile, adult onset)
Psychotic manifestations (1)	+					+		+	+	+		+	+	
Palpitations, insomnia anxiety, thin skin and nails				+										
Excess perspiration		+		+										
Weight gain		+				+				+				+
Weight loss				+					+			+		+
Loss of libido, amenorrhea	+	+												
Anorexia	+								+	+		+		
Asthenia (2)	+			+	+				+	+	+	+		+
Polydipsia, polyuria	+		+											+
Generalized edematous puffy features							+							
Nausea, vomiting						+			+	+		+		+
Sluggishness, sleepiness	+					+		+	+	+		+	+	
Severe headache	+	+						+						
Pruritus		+		+										
Peripheral neuropathy (3)		+				+						+		+
Ataxia, gait						+					+	+	+	+
Increased reflex time, hyporeflexia, areflexia						+								+
Decreased reflex time, hyperreflexia, hyperkinesis		+		+								+		
Arthralgia, bone pain, joint stiffness						+			+	+		+		+
Irritability, restlessness				+					+	+			+	+

Visual disturbances (impaired visual acuity)	+			+		+	+	+
Dysphagia						+		
Dyspnea on exertion	+				+	+		
Hypotension	+		+	+	+	+	+	
Hypertension						+		+
Argyll Robertson pupil			+			+		

anemia, iron deficiency anemia); *recurrent aphthous ulcers of the mouth* (agranulocytic angina, Crohn's disease); *pain on swallowing* may be localized, eg., substernal simulating angina pectoris; or *radiating burning sensation* (heartburn) related to reflux esophageal mucositis; *diaphragmatic* (hiatal) *hernia;* esophageal spasm, peptic ulcer disease; *gastritis* (gastropyrosis in iron deficiency anemia); *macroglossia, glossoptosis, atrophic papillae* (hyperthyroidism, endemic cretinism); *belching* (cholecystitis, dyspepsia); *hematemesis* (hiatal hernia, gastric, peptic ulcer disease, acute alcoholic hepatitis, carcinoma); *hemorrhage in the form of occult blood loss or melena* (GI carcinoma, hiatal hernia, peptic ulcer disease, ulcerative colitis, hemorrhoids); *steatorrhea* (chronic pancreatitis, mucoviscidosis of the pancreas); *diarrhea caused by chronic renal failure or specific infections* and inflammations of the intestine (cholera, shigellosis); *neoplasms* (colon carcinoma); irritable colon syndrome; sprue; food allergy and intolerance; thyrotoxicosis; neuropathy in uncontrolled diabetes mellitus; postgastrectomy; *cystic fibrosis* (mucoviscidosis) of the pancreas; *regional enteritis* (Crohn's disease); *granulomatous colitis* (Crohn's disease of the colon), ulcerative colitis, diverticulitis, gastritis); *flatulence* (cholecystitis, iron deficiency anemia, carcinoma of the pancreas); *borborygmus* (malabsorption); *nausea and vomiting* (acute cholecystitis, gastritis, gastroenteritis, hepatitis, acute alcoholic hepatitis, acute appendicitis, iron deficiency anemia, polycythemia, chronic pancreatitis, carcinoma of the pancreas, methemoglobinemia, peptic ulcer); *anorexia, weight loss* (chronic renal failure, malabsorption, carcinoma, chronic pancreatitis, acute cholecystitis, chronic active/aggressive hepatitis, regional enteritis, granulomatous enteritis, acute appendicitis); *abdominal distention* (chronic pancreatitis, tumor, ascites, cystic fibrosis of the pancreas, dyspepsia, malabsorption; *steady progressive, generalized abdominal pain, tenderness, discomfort* (carcinoma, dyspepsia, acute cholecystitis, acute alcoholic hepatitis, regional enteritis, granulomatous colitis, chronic active hepatitis, chronic leukemia, lymphoma, polycythemia, Addison's disease, hyperthyroidism, hypoparathyroidism, hyperparathyroidism); *recurrent attacks of severe abdominal pain, cramps* (acute viral hepatitis, fulminant hepatitis, chronic pancreatitis, cystic fibrosis of the pancreas); *chronic, severe, cramping* (characteristic mild to severe pain) localized at:

Lower abdomen (ulcerative colitis, malabsorption).

Periumbilical, epigastric area (malabsorption, lymphoma, gastroenteritis, acute pancreatitis, Zollinger-Ellison syndrome, peptic ulcer).

Lower left quadrant (diverticulitis).

Right lower quadrant—McBurney's point (acute appendicitis).

Right upper quadrant (cholecystitis, cholangitis, choledocholithiasis).

Radiating to the back in chronic pancreatitis.

Radiating to the subcostal region in cholangitis, choledocholithiasis.

Jaundice can be present in acute or chronic pancreatitis, acute viral hepatitis, chronic active (aggressive) hepatitis, acute alcoholic hepatitis; *constipation* (carcinoma of the pancreas, progressive systemic sclerosis, iron deficiency anemia, depression, myxedema, hyperparathyroidism, medications including opiates, anticholinergics, ganglionic blockers, antidepressants); *eating habits* (fast gulper, nibbler, slow); *enlargements* (lump of mass, asymmetry, gradual, rapid, painless or tender); *central obesity, rounding of the face, thick thoracicoabdominal panniculus* (Cushing's syndrome).

h. *Genitourinary:* Hematuria (renal cystic disease, glomerulonephritis, nephrolithiasis); *oliguria* (uremia, acute renal insufficiency, lymphoma, dehydration, diarrhea, obstructive nephropathy related to stone, prostate neoplasm, glomerulonephritis); *cloudy, foul smelling urine* (cystitis or pyelonephritis); *polyuria* with increased micturition urgency and frequency (cystitis, pregnancy, nervous excitement, nephritis, diabetes); *dysuria* or painful, difficult urination (renal cystic disease, diabetes mellitus, cystitis or pyelonephritis); *hypertension* (pyelonephritis, chronic renal failure, renal vascular disease, renal cystic disease, glomerulonephritis); *generalized edema* (glomerulonephritis, nephrotic syndrome, chronic renal failure or uremia); *renal colic or pain at lumbar, costovertebral areas* (renal cystic disease, hyperparathyroidism, nephrolithiasis, glomerulonephritis, pyelonephritis); *generalized fatigue, nausea, vomiting* (acute or chronic renal insufficiency, glomerulonephritis); *excessive bleeding, bruising* (chronic renal failure); *decreased resistance to infections* (candida albicans, staphyococcus superinfection in chronic renal disease), *dribbling, incontinence,* (lesion of the spinal cord lumbar center, relaxed sphincters); *urinary hesitancy* (difficulty starting stream as in urethral obstruction, eg., prostatism); *menstrual history:* (age of onset, or menarche, duration of cycle, amount of flow, regularity, date of last period); *oligomenorrhea* (Cushing's syndrome), *amenorrhea* (the absence of menstruation), *menorrhagia* or excessive menstrual bleeding (hypothyroidism), metrorrhagia (bleeding between periods often related to malignancy), *menopause* and the emotional reactions (permanent cessation of menstrual activity, subtotal or total hysterectomy) and associated hot flushes, disordered oral sensation, mental depression; *obstetrical history* (number of pregnancies, outcome, complications or abnormalities); *impotence* and diminished fertility (Cushing's syndrome, diabetes mellitus); *psychosis* (acute renal failure); *insomnia, areflexia, peripheral neuropathy, mental fatigability* (chronic renal failure).

i. *Hematopoietic* (see Table 1.2).

(1) Hemorrhage, spontaneous, excessive bleeding, easy bruising may be manifested as epistaxis, melena, menorrhagia, petechiae, ecchymoses, hematuria, hemarthroses, purpuric manifestations into the mucosae, skin, soft and hard tissues resulting in functional impairments, pain.

(2) Paresis, numbness, burning and tingling in the extremities, ataxia, unsteady gait, diminished reflexes.

(3) Prostration, tiredness, weakness, easy fatigability.

Additional clinical manifestations of hematologic disorders as to: methemoglobinemia (CNS depression), "megaloblastic madness" (paranoid ideation, depression, picture of paranoid schizophrenia, confusion, irritability, forgetfulness), iron deficiency anemia (irritability), hemochromatosis (impotence, peripheral neuropathy), polycythemia (lethargy, visual disturbances), acute hemolytic anemia (restlessness, syncope).

j. *Endocrine:* Hormone consumption (oral contraceptives); see Table 1.3.

(1) Psychologic abnormalities (psychosis, general mental deterioration, paranoia, mental confusion, delusion, mood changes, mania, depression, disorientation, emotional lability, impairment of memory, indifference to the surroundings, lethargy, "myxedema madness").

(2) Muscular weakness, fatigue, malaise, "pseudotabes diabetica."

(3) Paresthesia, anesthesia, hyperesthesia in extremities.

k. *Psychiatric and neurologic* (see Table 1.4 on neurologic disorders).

(1) Schizophrenia
(2) Paranoid schizophrenia
(3) Paranoia
(4) Manic-depressive psychosis
(5) Hysteria (malingering, Munchausen syndrome, hypochondriasis)
(6) Anxiety attack
(7) Metabolic encephalopathy (toxic psychosis, delirium)
(8) Dementia
(9) Parkinson's disease (paralysis agitans)
(10) Sydenham's chorea (rheumatic fever, encephalitis, hyperthyroidism, hypocalcemia, systemic lupus erythematosus)
(11) Huntington's chorea
(12) Cerebral transient ischemic attack
(13) Cerebral infarction
(14) Intracranial haemorrhage
(15) Brain abscess
(16) Cavernous sinus thrombosis
(17) Neurosyphilis
(18) Herpes zoster
(19) Herpes simplex encephalitis
(20) Anterior poliomyelitis
(21) Bulbar poliomyetitis
(22) Wernicke-Korsakoff syndrome
(23) Multiple sclerosis
(24) Epilepsy
(25) Intracranial neoplasm
(26) Peripheral neuropathy
(27) Brain trauma (concussion).

Table 1.4
Neurologic Disorders

	Disorientation in time, place, person, mental confusion, thinking errors, impaired memory (anterograde, retrograde amnesia), faulty judgment	Replies to questions which are off the point, either vague or unnecessarily detailed	Inclination to suicide, careless with money, jobs	Loss of care for basic physical needs, totally unaware of the situation	Cannot meet challenge, progressive deterioration of intelligence, dementia, disturbed problem solving, forgetful, cannot make a decision, a judgment, answer a question, follow problems, explain abstract words, concepts; unable to concentrate, dull mentation, uncertainty
1	+				+
2	+				
3	+				+
4	+				+
5					
6	+				+
7	+				+
8	+				+
9					
10					
11					
12					+
13					
14					+
15	+				
16					+
17	+				
18					+
19	+				
20					+
21					
22	+				+
23					+
24					
25	+				+
26					
27	+				+

Table 1.4—Continued

Emotional disturbances, fear, tears, easy and unpredictable anger, aggressiveness, hostility, irritability

No.		Description
1	+	Emotional unrest, disturbed emotional expression, seems distant, cold, incongruous, cries and laughs without reason, inappropriateness of mood
2	+	
3	+	Jealous, sensitive, megalomanic
4	+	Complains of feeling miserable, sadness, hopelessness, inadequacy, worthlessness, self-blame; or feeling of self-importance, excellent well-being, extreme confidence, running disconnected ideas, megalomania, euphoria
5		
6	+	Tension, extreme apprehension
7	+	
8	+	
9		
10	+	
11	+	
12		
13	+/−	
14	+/−	
15	+/−	
16		
17	+	
18		
19		
20		
21	+	
22	+	
23	+	
24		
25	+	
26		
27	+	

Table 1.4—Continued

Delusions

False beliefs, e.g., outside control of the thinking, the ill treatment is an underserved persecution
Suspiciousness and fear of mistreatment based on false beliefs
Fixed ideas developing into logical, systematized, progressive delusions of persecution, suspiciousness
Guilty delusions: the ill treatment is a justified punishment

#	Delusions	Anxiety	Insomnia	Depression, apathy, lethargy
1	+			
2	+			
3	+			
4	+			
5	+	+	+	+
6		+		+
7	+		+	
8	+	+	+	+
9				+
10				
11				
12				
13				+/−
14				+/−
15				+/−
16				+/−
17				+
18			+	+
19				
20		+		+
21				+
22				+/−
23			+	+
24				
25				+
26				+
27				+

Table 1.4—Continued

	Seizures, gross muscle contractions, multifocal myoclonus convulsions, tonic-clonic	Tremor, abnormal motor activity	Muscle weakness	Nausea, vomiting	Drowsiness	Muscle rigidity, immobility
1		+ Repetitive movements, facial grimaces				+ Maintaining unnatural posture
2						
3		+				
4		+ Energetic, extreme hyperactivity	+			
5	+ "Hysterical"	+ Ataxia				
6		+ Fine				
7	+	+ Irregular, coarse, extreme hyperactivity	+		+	+
8	+	+				
9		+ Rhythmic				+ Postural instability, stiffness of extremities, lack of facial expression, "mask face," akinesia or sudden arrest of action
10		+ Jerking, incoordination, purposeless, involuntary facial grimacing	+			
11		+ Jerking				
12		+ Ataxia	+ Unilateral	+		
13	+	+ Ataxia	+	+		+ Marked neck rigidity
14	+	+ Ataxia	+	+	+	+
15	+		+	+	+	+ Stiff neck, impaired coordination
16			+	+		
17	+	+ Tabes dorsalis or locomotive ataxia, broad-based gait				

Table 1.4—Continued

No.					Neurological features	
18				+		
19	+	+		+	Ataxia	
20		+		+	Ataxia	
21				+	Muscle cramps, twitching, fasciculations	
22	+		+	+	Ataxia	
23			+	+	Coarse tremor, incoordination, ataxia	
24	+	+	+	+	Ataxia	Cervical rigidity +
25	+		+	+		
26			+	+	Ataxia, gait, clumsiness	
27			+	+	Ataxia	

Table 1.4—Continued

	Delirium	Agitation, restlessness	Hallucinations, illusions	Confabulation	Lightheadedness, headache, dizziness, vertigo	Sensory disturbances (pain, neuralgia, paresthesia, somatic visceral tenderness, aches, prickling sensation, anesthesia)	Paralysis	Withdrawing, obtundation, stupor, clouding, unconsciousness	Anorexia, loss of weight, constipation	diarrhea
1			+ (Auditory)							
2	+		+ (Auditory)							
3		+	+			+			+	
4		+	+			+			+	
5				+	+	+ (Bizarre, unrelated to neuroauditory)	+	+		
6	+	+	+ (Frightening vivid nightmares)			+			+	+
7			+		+			+		
8										
9										
10										
11							+/−			
12					+ (Tinnitus)	+	+/− (Fleeting, contralateral to the ischemia)			
13	+				+	+	+ (Hemiparesis)	+/−		
14	+				+	+	+ (Contralateral or bilateral)	+/−		

Table 1.4—Continued

No.				Hemiparesis		Hemiplegia				
15	+								+/–	
16	+	+			Ophthalmoplegia					+/–	
17	+				Hemiparesis, delayed pain perception	+	Cranial nerve Hemiplegia	+	+	+	
18	+				Along the dermatome, postherpetic neuralgia, cranial nerve	+	Cranial nerve	+			
19	+		Olfactory, gustatory	+		+		+	+		
20	+	+			Myalgia	+	Flaccid	+	+	+	+
21	+	+				+	Cranial nerve	+			
22	+	+	+	+					+		
23	+	+	+			+		+	+		
24	+								+		
25	+	+				+		+	+	+	+
26	+				Trigeminal, glossopharyngeal, fingers, toes, face, oral cavity	+	Hemiplegia	+		+	
27	+						Ophthalmoplegia, Bell's palsy	+/–	+		

Table 1.4—Continued

	Abnormal speech, mutism, fluent, nonfluent aphasia	Visual impairment	Dysphagia	Incontinence	Deafness	Anosmia	Increased perspiration, xerostomia
1	+ "Schizophrenic word-salad"						
2							
3							
4	+		+		+		
5	+	"Hysterical blindness" +			+	+	+
6							
7	+						
8	+ Slurred speech						
9	+ Slow monotonous speech						
10	+ Difficulty in speech						
11		+	+				
12	+ Dysphonia, dysarthria	Blurred vision, diplopia +					
13	+ Dysphasia, dysarthria	Scotomas, diplopia +	+				
14	+	Hemianopia +					
15	+	Visual field defects, nystagmus +					
16		Photophobia, ophthalmodynia, periorbital edema +		+			
17		Hemianopia, Argyll Robertson pupil +	+				
18	+						
19	+	+					
20		+					
21	+						
22		Diplopia, nystagmus +					

Table 1.4—Continued

No.							Symptoms	
23			+		+			Diplopia
24							+	
25	+				+		+	Diplopia, dimming of vision, hemianopia, Argyll Robertson pupil
26	+	+	+	+			+	
27	+					+		Cranial nerves serving the speech organs; hoarseness

Examination Findings

LEVENTE Z. BODAK-GYOVAI

Once the historical data base is obtained one proceeds to obtain objective data by examining the patient. The examination is based on the recording of the objective signs and the associated subjective symptoms.

Careful clinical examination of the visible areas of the head, neck, extremities, and oral cavity during a routine dental checkup is reasonable to appraise the normal physical limits and to detect clinical manifestations of abnormalities, e.g., the presence of orofacial cancer in a high risk group of patients over 50 years of age.

In general, the most serious mistakes result from either the neglect to examine the patient or to follow systematic steps, rather than from failure to detect insignificant aberrations from the accepted norm. It is critical to master the simple methods of inspection, palpation, percussion and auscultation in a well organized pattern throughout the course of the examination, e.g., learn to make a "basic" examination of the oral cavity which is invariably performed in each new and recall visit patient.

Because the power of discrimination is dulled by fatigue, it is well to complete the examination relatively rapidly. The dentist, guided by data gathered from the health history, following a routine examination can essentially concentrate on the suggested particular diagnostic question. For example, the history of recent syphilis points to the need for careful examination of periodontal tissues, lips, regional lymph nodes and all the intraoral mucous membrane areas; it is also necessary to suspect every lesion site. Special sensory perception is supplemented by roentgenographs, pulp vitality tests and diagnostic laboratory procedures, e.g., the clinical observation of the tongue reveals changes suggestive of sideropenic anemia, and indicates the need for a microhematocrit reading, keeping in mind that the absence of tongue abnormalities does not rule out the presence of anemia and tongue changes are not exclusive of the anemia present.

Unlike the medical doctor, who usually carefully combines the review of systems with the thorough physical examination of all organ systems and anatomic regions, the dental doctor generally limits the clinical examination to the head, neck, the uncovered extremities, and the oral cavity.

Session One: Measurement of Vital Signs*

Values of normal physiologic functions of various organ systems are relative to the level of their cellular activity. Deviations from normal values of vital signs are influenced by both the degree of physical activity and pathologic disorder present; both are important measurable signs of the disease condition.

---

* To standardize the readings, register the vital signs of the patient at rest.

I. Temperature as Measured by Mouth

42,0 C	(107.6 F)	*fatal level*	
41.0 C	(105.8 F)	intense fever	
40.5 C	(104.9 F)	high fever	hyperthermia (pyrexia)
40.0 C	(104.0 F)	severe fever	
39.0 C	(102.2 F)	moderate fever	
38.0 C	(100.4 F)	slight fever	
37.0 C	(98.6 F)	*normal temperature*	
36.0 C	(96.8 F)	subnormal temperature	
34.0 C	(93.2 F)	cold collapse	hypothermia
26.0 C	(78.8 F)	*fatal level*	

It is essential that the patient abstain from hot food, smoking or cold beverages for about 10 minutes prior to oral temperature registration.

The median value of rectal temperature reading of an individual is about 0.5°C higher, the axillary (much used in Europe) is about 0.2°C lower than oral temperature. If septic, cyclic or sustained fever is recorded consider the circadian (diurnal) temperature variations: at 2 A.M. the axillary normal reading may be 36°C and 37.6°C at 2 P.M.

Some practical suggestions are:
   Shake the mercury level down in the thermometer.
   Measure for 10 minutes
   Record the reading.
   Reinsert for 1 more minute without shaking the thermometer.
   Make the final reading.

Some of the disease conditions related to hypothermia and hyperthermia are as follows.
   A. Hypothermia
      Heavy inebriation
      Delirium
      Debilitation
      Cachexia
      Blood dyscrasias (anemia, thrombocytopenia)
      Viral infections (which may cause leukopenia)
      Gastric perforation
      Hypothyroidism
   B. Hyperthermia
      Acute viral and bacterial infections
      Septicemias (the initial chills usually coincide with the microbial invasion and mark the onset of fever)
      Inflammation
      Acute leukemia
      Acute myocardial infarction
      Stressful exercise
      Hyperthyroidism

II. Respiratory Rate (RR)

The average, normal values are:
First year: 30 to 60 per minute.
Twenty-first:
      Male: 16 to 18 per minute.
      Female: 18 to 20 per minute.
Elderly: about 14 per minute.

To avoid voluntary activation of respiratory muscles in interference with resting consciousness it is essential to employ inconspicuous detection of RR.

The following conditions may affect respiratory rates.
   A. Hypoventilation
      Respiratory acidosis
      Metabolic alkalosis
      Drug intoxications (sedatives)
   B. Hyperventilation   (deep,   rapid breathing)
      Anxiety
      Emotional stress
      Delirious state
      Decreased partial pressure of oxygen as in high altitudes
      Pneumonia
      Pulmonary edema
      Respiratory alkalosis
      Uremia
      Hyperglycemic coma
      Metabolic acidosis
      Asthma
      Respiratory Infections
   C. Tachypnea (rapid, shallow breathing)
      Emotional stress
      Central nervous system defect (neurogenic)
      Unpleasant odor
      Strenuous exercise
      Hyperthermia

III. Pulse Rate (PR)

The average normal PR values are:
First year: 90 to 120 per minute.
Middle life: 60 to 75 per minute.
Elderly: 50 to 60 per minute.
   Bradycardia: PR is lower than 50 per minute, e.g., seen in aged.

Tachycardia: PR is higher than 100 per minute, e.g., fever, inflammation, organic heart disease, CNS lesion.

Determine pulse on both right and left sides, either central (carotid), or peripheral (radial). Count PR for 1 minute. Repeat if irregularity is encountered. Always record the character of the pulse by using three fingers (Figure 2.1) to note the following features (Table 2.1): Record complaints of

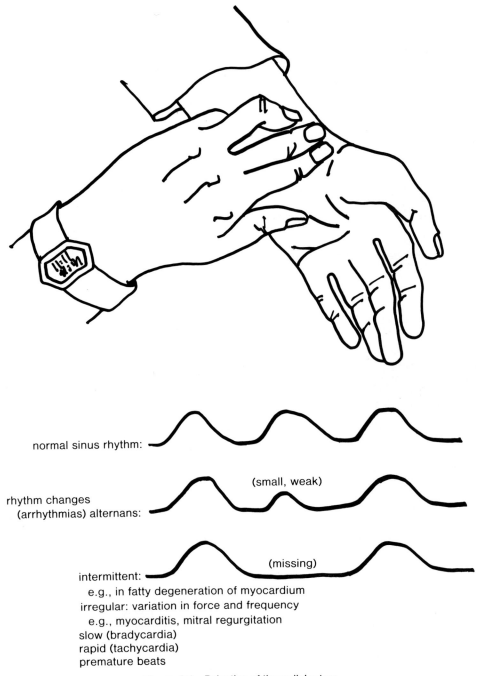

normal sinus rhythm:

(small, weak)

rhythm changes
(arrhythmias) alternans:

(missing)

intermittent:
  e.g., in fatty degeneration of myocardium
irregular: variation in force and frequency
  e.g., myocarditis, mitral regurgitation
slow (bradycardia)
rapid (tachycardia)
premature beats

Figure 2.1   Palpation of the radial artery.

Table 2.1
Pulse Characteristics

Normal sinus rhythm:
Rhythm changes (arrhythmias)
    Alternans:
    Intermittent:
        e.g., in fatty degeneration of myocardium
        Irregular: variation in force and frequency
        e.g., myocarditis, mitral regurgitation
    Slow (bradycardia)
    Rapid (tachycardia)
    Premature beats
    Pulsus bigeminus:
    Pulsus trigeminus:
    Dicrotic (notched):
        e.g., relaxed arteriolar musculature
High tension (durus) needs strong finger pressure to suspend the pulse:
        e.g., cardiomegaly due to myocardial hypertrophy
Low tension (mollis):
        e.g., cardiac decompensation
Thready (filiform):
Collapsing (bounding):
        e.g., decreased peripheral resistance
Small (parvus) ⎫
Late (tardus) ⎬ e.g. aortic stenosis
Long ⎭
Corrigan's, water hammer, jerky, pistol-shot:
        e.g., aortic insufficiency (regurgitation)

palpitations, duration of detected pulse change, and excise- or emotion-dependent pulse character.

Some examples of conditions related to pulse variations are:

A. Bradycardia (slow pulse rate)
    Convalescence
    Decreased metabolic rate (hypothyroidism, hypoadrenalism)
    Elevated cerebrospinal fluid pressure
    Medications (quinidine, digitalis)

B. Tachycardia (increased pulse rate)
    Emotional stress
    Strenuous exercise
    Hyperthermia (about 0.5°C per every 10 systoles)
    Anemia
    Severe hemorrhage
    Congestive heart failure
    Drug related sympathetic overtone (catecholamines, caffeine)
    Hyperthyroidism

The maximum accepted safe pulse rate with heavy physical exercise is about 200 systoles per minute minus the age of the patient in years.

IV. Systemic Arterial Blood Pressure (BP)

Any attempt to establish normal limits of arterial blood pressure (systolic per diastolic) is artificial. There are no definite age or sex standards to provide the proper reference point of blood pressure readings to a given individual to separate exactly the normal from high or low blood pressure. It is generally held that the basal blood pressure is the value obtained after 60 minutes rest in a supine position. The following values may indicate guidelines for BP measurement.

A. A healthy adult, from 105/80 to 145/95 mm Hg, having a difference between systolic and diastolic of 25 to 50 mm Hg at lower and upper limits, respectively.

B. Recorded average healthy adult systolic value is 126 ± 12 and the diastolic is 76 ± 10 mm Hg.

C. Less than 10% of physicians would accept a strict age relationship as:

	Systolic (mm Hg)	Diastolic (mm Hg)
Up to adolescence	90	60
Middle age	120	80
Elderly	140	90

D. Elevated blood pressure is presented as:
   Age 20 to 39 years: greater than 140/90 mm Hg.
   Age 40 to 59 years: greater than 150/95 mm Hg.
   Age 60 years and up: greater than 160/100 mm Hg.

E. The median value of relationship between both systolic and diastolic pressure (diastolic pressure plus one-third of pulse pressure) is used as a guide in normotensive patients: 90.0 (5.0 standard deviation), including:
   Age 34 years: 93.0 (8.0 standard deviation).
   Age 60 years: 89.5 (5.0 standard deviation).

The BP is highly labile: in normotensives there is an average 33 mm Hg systolic and 10 mm Hg diastolic diurnal variation of blood pressure: a decline during sleeping, a sharp rise at awakening, a more gradual rise during the active hours of the day, but a high increase during sharp stress. The diurnal variations are greater in hypertensives. A single BP reading indicating hypertension, particularly if the patient is in pain or having office related apprehension at the time of examination is quite unrepresentative of the average characteristic level of BP for the patient.

MEASUREMENT OF ARTERIAL BLOOD PRESSURE†

Blood pressure is an indirect index indicating the means by which body tissues are perfused with blood.

The auscultatory method employs the ordinary pressure cuff, the sphygmomanometer and the stethoscope (or phonendoscope).

The width of the cuff should be 20% higher than the diameter of the patient's arm.

Various cuff width sizes are available:
One year old's cuff: 2.5 cm standard width.
Children's cuff: 6.9 cm standard width.
Adult arm cuff: 12.0 cm standard width.
Obese adult arm (thigh) cuff: 18.0 cm standard width.

Some practical suggestion related to the reading of blood pressure are the following:

1. Determine the systolic blood pressure level by digital (palpatory) technique to avoid error at auscultatory gap.
2. Deflate the cuff pressure at the rate of 2 mm Hg per second.
3. Record diastolic pressure at the level when the Korotkoff sounds disappear and no longer can be detected.
4. Always record the nearest ever number (not like 135/69).
5. Allow 5 minutes rest by removing the blood pressure cuff.
6. Repeat the reading of systolic and diastolic again.
7. Record the lower blood pressure values of both readings in the patient's chart.

The auscultatory method is useful, but is far from being a precise technique for the following reasons.

1. The error of ± 8 mm Hg for both systolic and diastolic value is within normal limits.
2. By monitoring blood pressure on the extremities one cannot infer indications of the adequacy of blood perfusion of specific vital organ systems (brain, heart, liver, kidneys).
3. Considerable error can be attributed to the physical characteristics of the extremity: the size of the arm related to the width of the cuff, the length of the cuff (it should be at least 50 cm and completely encircle the arm), the position of the arm, and muscle tone.
4. The results can be influenced by the position of the patient, the presence of pain, ingested food, use of tobacco prior to monitoring of blood pressure, nervous tension, presence of sympathetic overtone (effect of vasocon-

---

† Right arm sitting (RASit) is recommended to standardize the office reading technique.

striction), tachypnea, arrhythmia, local environmental effects (personnel, climate).

5. Results can be influenced by failure to position the blood pressure cuff correctly over the artery, location of an outbulged cuff portion over the artery, inadequate rate of deflation of the blood pressure cuff, point of reading for the diastolic level, either when Korotkoff sounds are muffled or have disappeared.

The oscillometric blood pressure detection method employs a blood pressure cuff and a manometer registering the transmitted pulsation of the artery indicating the systolic and diastolic blood pressure.

Certain medical conditions induce *hypotension*, including cardiac decompensation, anemias, severe hemorrhage, convalescence from prolonged bed rest (postural or orthostatic hypertension), paralytic or bulbar poliomyelitis, adrenocortical insufficiency, hypothyroidism, malabsorption syndrome, collagen disorders, medications (CNS depressants, ganglionic blocking agents, vasodilators, etc.), which may develop into syncope, circulatory collapse and shock.

The pulse pressure (PP) is an absolute value of systolic blood pressure minus diastolic blood pressure level. The PP is considered to be within normal limits above 25 and below 50. The major significance of normal PP is in the blood perfusion pressure of the myocardium.

V. Height and Weight Measurement

For the purpose of daily routine dental office patient evaluation the simple visual diagnosis of obesity or underweight is sufficient. The precise determination of the nutritional status of the patient—as indicated by the question of a systemic disorder, including high arterial blood pressure, malnutrition, diabetes mellitus, or local (e.g., tongue) abnormality—can be quantitated by measuring height and weight (see Chapter 6).

Session Two: Examination of the Head, Neck and Oral Cavity

Thorough examination of the extraoral and intraoral structures is performed deliberately in an orderly sequence of steps to permit the examiner the maximum opportunity to detect all the abnormalities present. Inspection, palpation, percussion and auscultation are routine procedures in the clinical examination of the patient. The general examination of the dental patient should extend upon the integument, cranial nerves, head and neck lymph nodes, thyroid gland and laryngeal complex, nose, eyes, ears and temporomandibular joint, salivary glands, lips, buccal mucosa, vestibules, hard and soft palate, tongue, pharynx, floor of the mouth, gingivae, jaw bones and the alveoli, and the teeth.

Integument

The surface characteristics are related to symmetry, landmarks, integrity, shape, size, color, texture, consistency, tenderness and lesions.

The general inspection restricted to the exposed skin surfaces of the head, neck and extremities is usually adequate in a dental office. Hidden lesions behind the hairlines are searched for with care if indicated. If spectacles are worn they should be removed to permit unobstructed visualization of that area. Skin folds can be separated gently for open inspection. Excess cosmetics concealing a lesion of the skin, or the vermilion border of the lips need to be removed.

The normal anatomic landmarks, junctions, contours, asymmetries beyond normal, should be noted, i.e.: Increased abdominal girth (pregnancy, cirrhosis, right sided heart failure); *ankle edema* (varicose veins, right sided heart failure); *distended jugular veins* (right sided heart failure); *exophthalmos* (hyperthyroidism); *hand tremor* (hyperthyroidism, severe nervous tension, multiple sclerosis, paralysis agitans); noticeable pulsation of abnormally *tortuous temporal artery* (systemic arterial hypertension); functional integrity of muscles of *facial expression*; direction of *mandibular movements* during speech, and if possible, mastication; *motion of prominentia laryngea* during deglutition (tracheal tug); *limited movement* (stiffness) *of extremities*; intactness of voluntary *lingual movements*; *locomotive motions, spasticity, flaccid paralysis*; *limited vertebral functions*; *pattern of baldness, distribution of hair* (endocrinopathies); *hypertrichosis*, or *hirsutism* (due to pituitary, adrenal, or ovarian disorder); *patchy hair loss* (in alopecia areata, tineasis, trichotillomania, syphilis, chronic discoid lupus erythematosus, tuberculosis, leprosy), *diffuse hair loss* (in hypopituitarism, hypothyroidism, pneumonia, systemic lupus erythematosus, lymphomas, exfoliative dermatitis, dermatomyositis, excess vitamin A, antineoplastic agents); evidences of previous skin *traumas*; involuntary *head movements* (tremor indicating neuromuscular disorder, or primary central nervous system lesion; clubbed *finger nails* (cardiopulmonary disorder).

The characteristic appearance of the *face can be mask-like, taut* (scleroderma); *moon-shaped* (Cushing's disease, or syndrome); *leonine* (Paget's disease of bone, leprosy); *puffy and myxedematous* (hypothyroidism); *sardonic* (paralysis, risus sardonicus in tetanus); *anxious* (stress, depression, hyperthyroidism, predelirium tremens); *flushed* (alcoholism, systemic arterial hypertension, chronic febrile disorders, e.g., pulmonary tuberculosis); *asymmetry, deformities and swellings* of the jaws (dental and nondental causes); *relaxed neutral* face (Parkinson's disease); *sunken* features (cachexia in terminal malignancy or wasting advanced pulmonary tuberculosis; pituitary atrophy).

The skin color changes, like *cyanosis* or *blueness* (cardiopulmonary disease, local stasis with unsaturated hemoglobin, polycythemia); *redness* (fever, hyperthyroidism, rule out vascular neoplasms, hemangiomas by diascopic blanching, detection of pulsation); *yellowness* (jaundice, carotenemia); *pallor* (may also be seen on the conjunctivae in anemia, severe stress or shock and circulatory collapse related to vascular insufficiency, albinism); *bluish fingernails* (pulmonary or cardiac decompensation).

The *pathologic signs* including erythema, various forms of exanthems, eruptions, or rash, e.g., macula, papula, pustula, vesicle, bulla, erosion, ulcer, crusting, scaling, scars, atophy, pigmentation, petechiae, ecchymoses, vibex, purpura may be seen.

One must employ *palpation* of texture, elasticity, moisture (severe apprehension, anxiety), muscle tone, tenderness, masses (soft, movable, fluctuant, indurated, fixed,

localized nodules, diffuse swellings), temperature (palpate with the dorsal surface of the hand or use the middle phalanges), sensory functions, numbness, employ diascopy to examine surface localized soft tissue lesions (telangiectases, lupus vulgaris, localized phlebectasia).

Other routine procedures include percussion of jaw fracture regions, sinus areas and teeth, and auscultation for thyroid bruit or "thrill" of very vascular hyperthyroid gland, crepitus of temporomandibular joint, premature tooth occlusion and bruxism.

ELEMENTARY DERMATOLOGIC LESIONS

Primary dermatologic lesions are the following:
1. Macule (Figure 2.2)
   Less than 10 mm in diameter.
   Flat.
   E.g., melanotic freckles, nevi.
2. Patch (Figure 2.3)
   More than 10 mm in diameter.
   Flat.
   E.g., port-wine nevus, measles, vitiligo, senile freckles, melasma, chloasma.
3. Papule (Figure 2.4)
   Less than 10 mm in diameter.
   Elevated.
   E.g., lichen planus, nevi, warts, verruca vulgaris, nummular eczema, wheals of insect bites and hives.

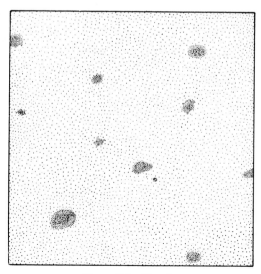

Figure 2.2 Macules.

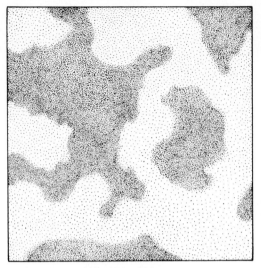

Figure 2.3   Patches.

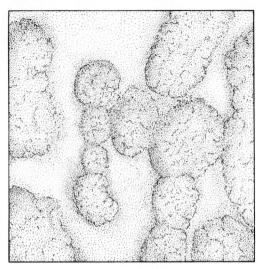

Figure 2.5   Plaques.

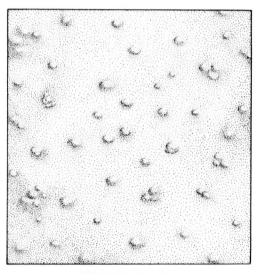

Figure 2.4   Papules.

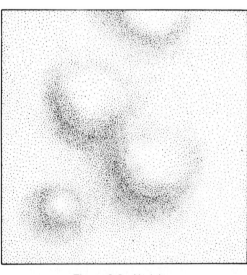

Figure 2.6   Nodules.

4. Plaque (Figure 2.5)
   More than 10 mm in diameter.
   Elevated.
   E.g., sarcoidosis, mycosis fungoides.
5. Nodule (Figure 2.6)
   Less than 10 mm in diameter.
   Elevated or depressed.
   E.g., epithelioma, xanthoma, tertiary syphiloderm, tuberculosis cutis verrucosa, keloid.
6. Tumor (Figure 2.7)
   More than 10 mm in diameter.
   Elevated or depressed.
   E.g., benign or malignant neoplasms.

7. Vesicle (Figure 2.8)
   Less than 10 mm in diameter.
   Serous content.
   E.g., herpes simplex, herpes zoster, varicella, dermatitis venenata, pemphigus.
8. Bulla (Figure 2.9)
   More than 10 mm in diameter.
   Serous content.
   E.g., burns, pemphigus, bullous lichen planus.
9. Pustule (Figure 2.10)
   Different sizes.
   Purulent content.

E.g., impetigo contagiosa, acne vulgaris, pustular psoriasis.

10. Petechia (Figure 2.11)

   Less than 10 mm in diameter.

   Content of blood elements.

   E.g., dermatitis venenata or medicamentosa, vascular, clotting or platelet disorders, insect bites, avitaminosis C.

11. Purpura (Figure 2.12)

   More than 10 mm in diameter.

   Content of blood elements.

   E.g., hemophilia, senile purpura, vascular, clotting or platelet disorders.

Secondary dermatologic lesions are the following:

1. Scale (squama, exfoliation) (Figure 2.13)

   Dry or oily desquamation of the circumscribed superficial portion of epithelium.

   E.g., psoriasis, dandruff.

2. Crust (scab) (Figure 2.14)

   Circumscribed.

   Elevated.

   Discolored exudate.

   E.g., impetigo contagiosa.

3. Excoriation (erosion, abrasion) (Figure 2.15)

   Circumscribed.

   Depressed.

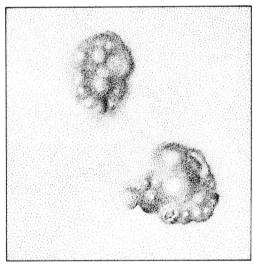

Figure 2.7 Tumors.

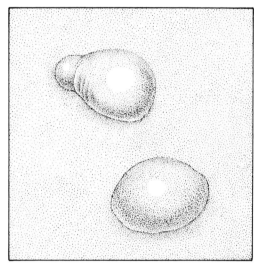

Figure 2.9 Bullae.

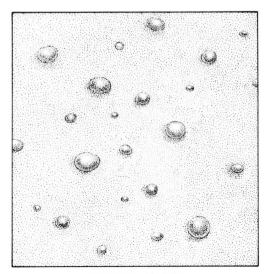

Figure 2.8 Vesicles.

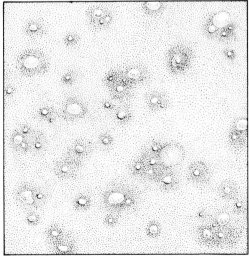

Figure 2.10 Pustules.

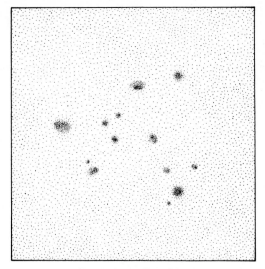

Figure 2.11   Petechiae.

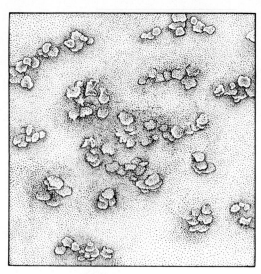

Figure 2.13   Scales.

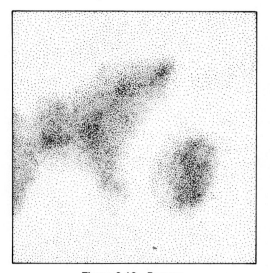

Figure 2.12   Purpura.

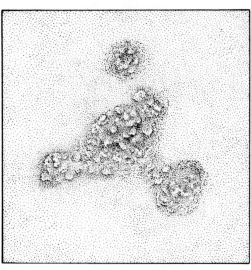

Figure 2.14   Crusts.

Discolored.
E.g., scabies, scratched eruptions, neurodermatitis.
4. Fissure (Figure 2.16)
Linear, sharply demarcated.
Depressed.
E.g., syphilis, tinea pedis.
5. Ulcer (ulcus) (Figure 2.17)
Circumscribed.
Depressed.
E.g., decubitus, syphilis, cancer.
6. Scar (cicatrix) (Figure 2.18)
Circumscribed.
Elevated.
E.g., keloid (hypertrophic scar).

7. Lichenification (Figure 2.19)
Patches of scaly, dry, thickened epithelium.
E.g., neurodermatitis.
In general the primary dermatologic lesions are obscured by secondary characters resulting in combinations of signs.:
1. Papulosquamous lesions (Figure 2.20)
E.g. tinea versicolor, secondary syphilis, psoriasis, pityriasis rosea.
2. Crusted excoriations
E.g. infected dermatitis, seborrheic dermatitis.

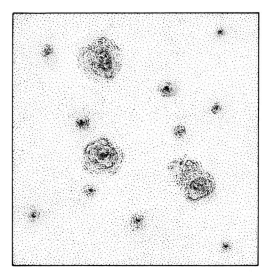

Figure 2.15 Excoriations (some crusted).

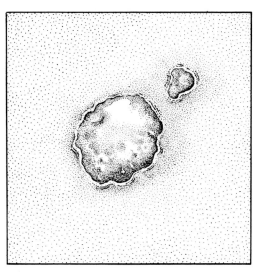

Figure 2.17 Ulcers.

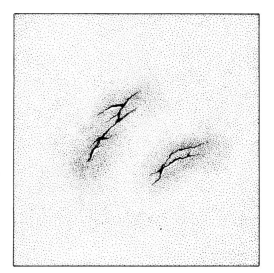

Figure 2.16 Fissures.

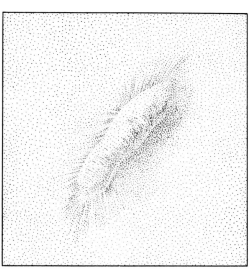

Figure 2.18 Scar.

3. Vesiculopustular lesions (Figure 2.21)
   E.g. dermatitis venenata.

Specialized dermatologic lesions

1. Acne (comedones, blackheads) (Figure 2.22)
   Small, circumscribed, elevated plug in the pilosebaceous follicle.
2. Milia (whitehead) (Figure 2.23)
   Less than 2 mm in diameter.
   Elevated.
   Superficial.
3. Burrow (Figure 2.24)
   Intraepidermal tunnel.
   E.g., scabies.

4. Telangiectasia (Figure 2.25)
   Superficial vasodilation.
   E.g., hereditary hemorrhagic telangiectasis, radiodermatitis, spider hemangioma.

The following relatively common *dermatologic lesions* will be described briefly according to the etiology involved.

BACTERIAL DERMATITIS

A. Pyoderma (primary bacterial dermatitis). Etiologic agents: coagulase positive staphylocci; β hemolytic streptococci (streptococcus pyogenes)

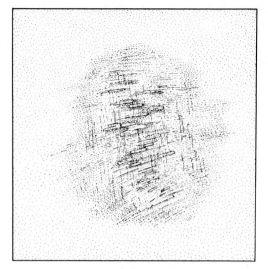

Figure 2.19   Lichenification.

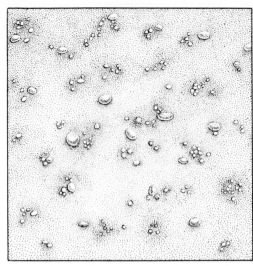

Figure 2.21   Vesiculopustular lesions.

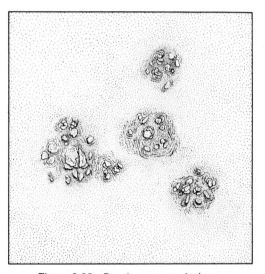

Figure 2.20   Papulosquamous lesions.

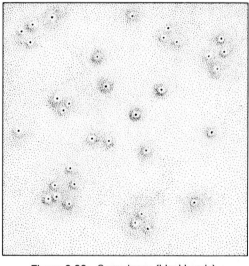

Figure 2.22   Comedones (blackheads).

1. Folliculitis: minor infection of the hair follicle which can extend to the hair bulb. Usually chronic, recurrent, pruritic, pustular lesions. Scratching results in crusts of various sizes and depths in which case the involvement of the adjacent connective tissue region causes scars with atrophic centers. Areas commonly involved are the scalp, neck, face, eyelids (stye or hordeolum), chest and arms.

Differential diagnosis: contact dermatitis, chronic discoid lupus erythematosus, tinea.

Treatment: (a) topical dermatologic medications, depilation; (b) systemic antibiotics; (c) rule out systemic disorder.

2. Furuncle (boil): extensive infection of a single hair follicle.

Differential diagnosis: drug allergy, syphilis, tuberculosis, anthrax, blastomycosis, coccidioidomycosis, sporotrichosis, tularemia.

Treatment: (a) Rule out systemic involvement, e.g., diabetes mellitus, focus of infection in teeth, tonsils, gallbladder, genitourinary tract, etc; (b) topical dermatologic preparations; (c) incision and drainage; (d) parenteral antibiotics.

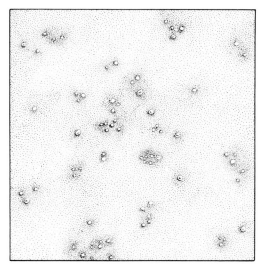

Figure 2.23 Milia (whiteheads).

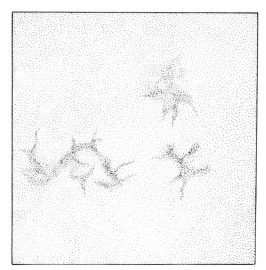

Figure 2.25 Telangiectasia.

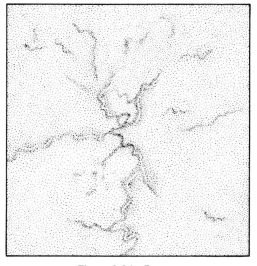

Figure 2.24 Burrows.

3. Carbuncle: several adjoining furuncles with multiple draining sinuses. Treatment is the same as for the furuncle.

4. Apocrinitis: infection of a single sweat gland, usually in the axilla. Treatment is the same as for the furuncle.

5. Hidradenitis suppurativa: chronic recurring, multiple abscesses of the adjoining sweat glands with draining sinuses. Commonly in the axilla.

Treatment: (a) incision and drainage; (b) systemic antibiotics; (c) topical dermatologic agents.

6. Erysipelas: β hemolytic streptococcus infection of the subcutaneous tissue. Sharply demarcated, spreading, reddening, painful plaque which may exhibit vesicles and bullae.

Differential diagnosis: cellulitis, contact dermatitis.

Treatment: (a) topical dermatologic medications; (b) systemic antibiotics.

7. Impetigo contagiosa: vesicles and bullae appearing in crops which became pustular, discharged and thin crusted.

Differential diagnosis: contact dermatitis, tinea.

Treatment: (a) topical dermatologic medication; (b) systemic antibiotic.

B. Secondary bacterial dermatitis. Picture of a primary dermatologic condition infected by pathogenic bacteria, usually streptococci or staphylococci.

1. Infected ulcers: Primary ulcers are seen in cancer and specific infections, including fungi, anthrax, leprosy, tuberculosis, clostridia, syphilis, etc. Secondary ulcers are signs of thrombosis, Raynaud's syndrome, arteriosclerosis, phlebitis, thromboangiitis obliterans, diabetes mellitus, traumatic (decubitus) ulcer, ulcerative colitis, phagedenic (spreading slough), peripheral vascular disease.

Treatment: (a) local dermatologic medications; (b) systemic antibiotics; (c) bed rest.

2. Infectious eczematoid dermatitis: widespread vesicles, oozing vesiculopustulous plaques with crusting and scaling.

Differential diagnosis: infected contact dermatitis, seborrheic dermatitis, nummular eczema.

Treatment: (a) local dermatologic preparations; (b) systemic antibiotics; (c) corticosteroids.

3. Bacterial intertrigo: friction of skin fold, heat and sweat result in red, macerated, patch. Predisposing factors: diabetes mellitus, obesity, personal hygiene related to urine, feces and menstruation.

Differential diagnosis: monilial intertrigo, tinea, seborrheic dermatitis.

Treatment: (a) topical dermatologic medications; (b) scrupulous personal hygiene.

4. Cutaneous diseases with secondary bacterial infection, e.g., contact dermatitis, fungal infection, traumatic abrasion, radiodermatitis.

C. Dermatitis in systemic bacterial infection.

1. Tuberculosis: formation of tuberculous skin granulomas caused by Mycobacterium tuberculosis.

    a. Tuberculosis chancre: primary complex related to the skin and regional lymph node.

    b. Miliary tuberculosis: primary hematogenous dissemination.

    c. Lesions developing in tuberculin positive patient (had previous tuberculous infection). Lupus vulgaris: extending area of plaques, nodules, ulcers, and scarring. Scrofuloderma: discharge from a subcutaneous focus (lymph node, bone). Tuberculosis cutis orificialis: involvement of mucocutaneous junction. Tuberculosis cutis verrucosa: wart-like formations.

Differential diagnosis: neoplasms, fungal infections, syphilis, leprosy, lupus erythematosus, sarcoidosis.

Treatment: antibacterial medications, including isonicotinic acid, para-aminosalicyclic acid, streptomycin.

2. Leprosy: granulomas develop due to Mycobacterium leprae. Lepromatous leprosy: infiltrated, progressive reddish macules, indefinite borders. Tuberculoid leprosy: erthematous area with elevated, sharp borders and central atrophy; associated with some degree of anesthesia.

Differential diagnosis: tuberculosis, syphilis, fungal infections, sarcoidosis.

Treatment: diaminodiphenyl sulfone, diazone.

3. Chancroid: caused by Haemophilus ducreyi. The primary lesion is an erosion surrounded by an erythematous, edematous halo. The secondary lesion is a gangrenous ulcer. There is prominent regional lymphadenopathy which may suppurate and form sinuses.

Differential diagnosis: syphilis, lymphogranuloma venereum, herpes simplex progenitalis, granuloma inguinale.

Treatment: tetracycline, sulfonamides.

4. Granuloma inguinale: due to Calymmatobacterium granulomatis. Formation of irregular superficial, bright red ulcer which heals by scarring.

Differential diagnosis: squamous cell carcinoma, primary syphilis, chancroid, granuloma pyogenicum.

Treatment: dihydrostreptomycin, oxytetracycline.

5. Scarlet fever: caused by streptococcal infection resulting in small, confluent macular eruptions first on the central part of the body and spreads centrifugally leaving a perioral pallor.

Differential diagnosis: measles, drug allergy.

Treatment: antibiotics.

6. Syphilis: due to Treponema pallidum.

    a. Primary syphilitic chancre: single (or multiple) indurated ulcer with sharp borders and surrounding edema. Healing is usually unremarkable. Regional lymphadenopathy persists.

    b. Sedondary syphilis: nonpruritic syphilitic rash involves the entire skin surface exhibiting macules, papules, pustules, erosions, flat and warty lesions (condylomata lata), nodules and ulcerations at various developmental stages, configurations and combinations, e.g., papulosquamous, crusted excoriations, maculosquamous, pustulonodular. Patchy alopecia of the scalp and annular lesions of the face are typical.

    c. Tertiary syphilis: annular, and nodular lesions, gummatous ulcerations, scarring, perforation on healing, e.g., soft palate, Charcot joint.

   d. Congenital syphilis: clinical manifestations are usually those of secondary syphilis.

Differential diagnosis: chancroid, herpes simplex, fungal infections, tuberculosis, leprosy, sarcoidosis, neoplasms.

Treatment: antibiotics.

VIRAL DERMATITIS

A. Measles (rubeola, morbilli). Typical Koplik spots around the parotid papillae and on the lower lip; bluish maculae or erythematous base. The morbilliform rash begins on the head, extends through the neck, chest and extremities; consists of reddish patches, papules; scales upon healing.

Differential diagnosis: scarlet fever, German measles, drug allergy, infectious mononucleosis.

Treatment: vaccine prophylaxis.

B. German measles (rubella). The eruption spreads in the same manner as in measles, the redness is milder, and typical postauricular, cervical lymphadenopathy is present.

Differential diagnosis: measles, scarlet fever, drug allergy.

Treatment: vaccine prophylaxis.

C. Chickenpox (varicella). Small vesicles appearing on the trunk and spreading centrifugally. New crops of vesicles appear for a few days. Pustules and crusts develop. Pruritus is prominent.

Treatment: local dermatologic preparations.

D. Shingles (herpes zoster). Usually unilateral (rarely bilateral) multiple groups of small vesicles following the distribution of a nerve. New crops of vesicles appear for a few days. Pustules, ulcers, crusts develop; may cause scarring. Postherpetic pain is characteristic.

Differential diagnosis: herpes simplex.

Treatment: (a) topical dermatologic medications; (b) analgesics.

E. Herpes simplex
   1. Primary herpes simplex: prominent constitutional signs and symptoms and appearance of single group of small vesicles (fever blisters). Pain is moderate.

   2. Recurrent herpes simplex: group of small vesicles which develop into erosions and crusts. Recurrences are localized, e.g., lips, genitalia, eyes (corneal dendritic ulcer, marginal keratitis), mouth.

Differential diagnosis: recurrent aphthous stomatitis, herpes zoster, tinea, syphilis.

Treatment: symptomatic.

F. Kaposi's varicelliform eruption. Appears in child with atopic eczema autoinoculated with herpes simplex or vaccinia virus. Generalized distribution of small umbilicated vesicles.

Treatment: supportive.

G. Wart (verruca).
   1. Common wart (verruca vulgaris): papillary, circumscribed growth.
   2. Moist wart (condylomata acuminata): soft verrucous mass.
   3. Plantar wart: single or multiple flat lesions may coalesce into mosaic pattern.
   4. Filiform wart: fingerlike projections.

Differential diagnosis: seborrheic keratosis, nonpigmented verrucous nevus, callus formation, cutaneous horn, pedunculated fibroma.

Treatment: (a) local dermatologic preparations; (b) electrosurgery.

FUNGAL DERMATITIS

A. Tinea. Ringworm is caused by *Microsporum*, *Epidermophyton*, *Trichophyton* or ectothrix. The location of infection is the feet (tinea pedis), hands (tinea manus), nails (onychomycosis), trunk (tinea corporis), groin (tinea cruris), external ear (otitis externa), scalp (tinea capitis), beard (tinea barbae). Small vesicles develop on the erythematous area, annoying pruritus, oozing of serous fluid, formation of dry scaly lesions of various shapes and sizes. The borders are sharp. The lesion may exhibit lichenification. In case of onychomycosis no vesicles are present, nail detachment and thickened deformity are noticed. In case of tinea capitis the noninflammatory type is characterized by grayish scaly, dry, crusted patches with hair loss. The inflammatory type presents follicular, pustular, scaly patches with hair loss. The hair regenerates following treatment,

Differential diagnosis: alopecia areata, seborrheic dermatitis, psoriasis, trichotillomania, pyoderma, contact dermatitis, atopic eczema, moniliasis, prickly heat, neurodermatitis and impetigo.

Treatment: (a) antifungal dermatologic preparations; (b) oral antimycotics (Griseofulvin, Grisactin, Grifulvin).

B. Tinea versicolor. Due to *Malassezia furfur*, exhibiting tan colored maculopapulosquamous polygonal, scaly patches.

Differential diagnosis: syphilis, seborrheic dermatitis.

Treatment: local dermatologic medications.

C. Moniliasis. Caused by *Candida albicans*.
  1. Monilial intertrigo: red eroded patches, vesiculopustulous, pustulous, scaly, diffuse lesions of skin fold areas.
  2. Monilial paronychia: red painful edematous periungual area.
  3. Generalized cutaneous moniliasis: involves any of the skin surfaces of a debilitated patient.
  4. Perlèche: cracks or fissures at the corners of the mouth, red base, crusts.

Differential diagnosis: allergic dermatitis, tinea, seborrheic dermatitis.

Treatment: topical antimycotic preparations.

D. Actinomycosis. *Actinomyces israelii* causes red, painless, firm granulomatous lesion usually in the jaw region (lumpy jaw) with pus discharging sinuses.

Differential diagnosis: neoplasms, pyoderma, tuberculosis.

Treatment: antibiotics.

E. North American blastomycosis. Due to *Blastomyces dermatitidis*. Primary chancre develops at the site of inoculation along regional lymphadenopathy. Secondary skin involvement appears in systemic infection: papule, pustule, ulcer with warty raised border.

Differential diagnosis: neoplasms, tuberculosis, syphilis, allergic dermatitis, pyoderma.

Treatment: amphotericin B.

F. Sporotrichosis. Caused by *Sporotrichum schenkii*. Painless soft granuloma, a freely movable subcutaneous module that develops into an ulcer. May form a chain of ulcers along the draining lymphatic vessel.

Differential diagnosis: leprosy, tuberculosis, sarcoidosis, syphilis, pyoderma.

Treatment: potassium iodide preparation, p.o.

PARASITIC DERMATOSES

A. Pediculosis. Lice insect infestation of hair (*Pediculus capitis*), body (*Pediculus corporis*), pubic area (*phthirus pubis*) results in itching, red, linear excoriations, morbilliform eruption. Regional lymphadenopathy.

Differential diagnosis: pyoderma, seborrheic dermatitis, scabies.

Treatment: topical dermatologic preparations.

B. Scabies. Extensive burrows are caused by the mite *Sarcoptes scabiei* resulting in generalized excoriated eruptions due to intense pruritus and scratching. Vesicles over burrows are seen.

Differential diagnosis: pyoderma, pediculosis, dermatitis herpetiformis.

Treatment: topical dermatologic preparations.

C. Helminthiasis. Due to roundworms (ancylostomiasis), or flatworms (schistosomiasis). The lesions are pruritic creeping eruptions, vesicles, papules over the burrows.

D. Leishmaniasis. Due to *Leishmania braziliensis*. The mucocutaneous form is characterized by multiple nodules with painful ulcers, necrosis. The cutaneous form (oriental sore) is ulcerated, crusted lesions with rolled border.

Differential diagnosis: fungal infections, neoplasms, syphilis.

Treatment: amphotericin B.

ALLERGIC DERMATITIS

A. Drug eruption (dermatitis medicamentosa) is caused by any systematically administered (per os or parenteral) medication. The presented lesions include generalized erythematous, maculopapular eruption, urticaria, purpura, vesicles or bullae, exfoliative changes, pruritus, lichenification.

Differential diagnosis: erythema multiforme, photosensitivity reaction, exfoliative dermatitis, lichen planus, pemphigus, systemic disorders leading to purpric lesions, seborrheic dermatitis, eczematous eruptions, measles, scarlet fever.

Treatment: (a) discontinue any medication; (b) corticosteroids.

B. Contact dermatitis (dermatitis venenata) is eruption due to allergy (or irritation) from locally applied medication or substance, e.g., soaps, cosmetics, metals, toothpaste: erythema, edema, vesicles, bullae with oozing, crusting, pruritus, excoriations, exfoliation, and lichenification.

Differential diagnosis: eczematous dermatitis.

Treatment: (a) local dermatologic preparations; (b) elimination of the etiologic factor.

C. Atopic eczema. Due to heredity, emotional stress, food allergy, dryness of the skin resulting in lichenification, xeroderma, pruritus, excoriations and exfoliation.

Differential diagnosis: contact dermatitis, psoriasis, neurodermatitis.

Treatment: (a) local dermatologic preparations; (b) corticosteroids.

D. Nummular eczema. Due to constitutional predisposition to allergies (asthma, hay fever), pyoderma, dry skin. The lesions are coin-shaped papulovesicular patches with lichenification.

Differential diagnosis: contact dermatitis, atopic eczema, psoriasis.

Treatment: (a) local dermatologic preparations, (b) dietary recommendations.

DERMATOSES CAUSED BY UNKNOWN ETIOLOGIC FACTORS

A. Seborrheic dermatitis, or dandruff is a skin condition, part of the "acne-seborrhea complex": erythematous patches with dry or greasy scaling, pruritus and excoriations, lichenification.

Differential diagnosis: lupus erythematosus, atopic eczema, tinea, psoriasis, neurodermatitis.

Treatment: (a) local dermatologic preparations; (b) personal hygiene.

B. Acne vulgaris; characterized by blackheads (comedones), papules, pustules, (cysts), excoriations and pitting scars.

Differential diagnosis: contact dermatitis, drug eruption.

Treatment: (a) personal hygiene; (b) local dermatologic preparations; (c) correction of hormonal imbalance; (d) improve general health and nutrition.

C. Rosacea: Erythematous areas with papules, pustules; may result in rhinophyma (hypertrophic nose).

Differential diagnosis: pyoderma, drug eruption, seborrheic dermatitis.

Treatment: (a) correction of diet (including abuse of alcohol); (b) local dermatologic preparations.

D. Psoriasis: family history is often positive, frequently seen in poststreptococcal sore throat infections (acute form, or guttate psoriasis). Chronic erythematous areas with silvery papulosquamous scaly lesions which bleed upon removal (Auspitz sign), excoriations, oozing and lichenification. Areas of usual skin injury are most affected (Köbner phenomenon).

Differential diagnosis: lichen planus, seborrheic dermatitis, tinea, syphilis, neurodermatitis, atopic eczema.

Treatment: local dermatologic preparations.

E. Pityriasis rosea: erythematous, rounded solitary papulosquamous lesions with pruritus, developing usually along the cleavage lines. A solitary "herald patch" may precede the general eruption.

Differential diagnosis: lichen planus, seborrhea dermatitis, psoriasis, syphilis, drug eruption, tinea.

Treatment: topical dermatologic preparations.

F. Lichen planus: purplish flat papules, papulosquamous pruritic lesions, chronic course.

Differential diagnosis: drug eruption, psoriasis, syphilis, pityriasis rosea.

Treatment: (a) local dermatologic medications; (b) systemic corticosteroids.

G. Neurodermatitis: red dry, scaly, pruritic patch, excoriations, lichenification.

Differential diagnosis: contact dermatitis, psoriasis, lichen planus, seborrheic dermatitis, atopic eczema.

Treatment: (a) local dermatologic medications; (b) tranquilizers.

H. Urticaria: rule out allergy to penicillin, foods, insect bites, cold, heat, inhalant allergens, rheumatic fever, liver involvement, neoplasms, local infections. Hives are characterized by papules of various sizes and shapes with red margins and white centers.

Treatment: (a) local dermatologic medications; (b) systemic corticosteroids; (c) sedatives, tranquilizers.

I. Erythema multiforme: red iris-shaped macules, papules, bullae, purpura, ulcers and associated fever, pruritus, arthralgia. Variations of this disease are:

1. Stevens-Johnson syndrome (ophthalmic and mucocutaneous involvement).
2. Behcet's syndrome (ophthalmic and mucocutaneous, mainly oral and genital lesions).
3. Reiter's syndrome (ophthalmic, mucosal and arthritic form).
4. Erythema multiforme bullosum.

J. Stasis dermatitis. Red, pruritic, scaly patch, vesicle, ulcer, crust, edema.

Differential diagnosis: neurodermatitis, contact dermatitis.

Treatment: (a) bed rest; (b) systemic antibiotics; (c) topical dermatologic preparations.

K. Pemphigus vulgaris: rubbing the skin produces moist surface (Nikolsky sign), vesicles, bullae develop that rupture, leaving eroded surfaces, crusts. The variations are erythematous, crusted, eroded lesions (pemphigus erythematosus), vegetations, granulomatous masses (pemphigus vegetans), scaly, moist exfoliations (pemphigus foliaceus).

Differential diagnosis: dermatitis herpetiformis, erythema multiforme bullosum, contact dermatitis, drug eruption, photosensitivity reaction of porphyria.

Treatment: (a) systemic corticosteroids; (b) topical dermatologic medications.

L. Dermatitis herpetiformis: papular, vesicular pruritic lesions, excoriations and hyperpigmentation.

Differential diagnosis: pemphigus, scabies, neurodermatitis.

Treatment: (a) local antipruritics; (b) systemic sulfa drugs, corticosteroids.

M. Vitiligo: progressive polygonal depigmented patches.

Differential diagnosis: albinism, tinea, lupus erythematosus, scleroderma, psoriasis, pinta, syphilis, hormonal disorders, nonpigmented nevus, medications.

Treatment: Oxsoralen, Trisoralen.

N. Chloasma: irregular, progressive melanin hyperpigmented areas.

Differential diagnosis: hyperthyroidism, pregnancy, Addison's disease, chronic liver disease, Peutz-Jeghers syndrome, Albright syndrome, acanthosis nigricans, Fanconi's syndrome, hormone administration, radiation therapy, excess ultraviolet radiation, systemic lupus erythematosus.

Treatment: topical dermatological preparations.

O. Lupus erythematosus.
1. Chronic, discoid lupus erythematosus is characterized by red, exfoliative patches with elevated borders, central atrophy, scarring, hypo- or hyperpigmentation, permanent hair loss of the affected area.

Differential diagnosis: sarcoidosis, syphilis, lupus vulgaris, systemic lupus erythematosus, seborrheic dermatitis, actinic dermatitis.

Treatment: (a) antimalarial medications; (b) topical dermatologic preparations.

2. Systemic lupus erythematosus exhibits red, exfoliative diffuse patches.

Differential diagnosis: contact dermatitis, actinic dermatitis, seborrheic dermatitis, drug eruption, chronic discoid lupus erythematosus.

Treatment: corticosteroids.

P. Scleroderma.
1. Localized scleroderma (morphea) presents inelastic, violaceous macules with whitish atrophic center, scarring, slow enlargement.

Differential diagnosis: lichen planus, traumatic scars.

2. Diffuse scleroderma presents progressive fixation of the skin, atrophy, melanin hyperpigmentation, ulcerations.

Differential diagnosis: dermatomyositis.

Treatment: symptomatic.

Q. Sarcoidosis: violaceous, reddish, polygonal papules, nodules, plaques with central atropy and scarring.

Differential diagnosis: syphilis, tuberculosis, lupus erythematosus, leprosy.

Treatment: (a) corticosteroids; (b) calciferol.

DERMATOSES IN INTERNAL DISEASES

A. Diabetes mellitus: tineasis, pyodermas, pruritus, xanthomas.

B. Hyperthyroidism: seborrhea, acne, moist erythematous hyperpigmented skin.

C. Hypothyroidism: coarse, dry, scaly, cool hyperpigmented skin.

D. Acromegaly: coarse, oily, hyperpigmented skin, increased sweating.

E. Cushing's syndrome: pyodermas, violaceous atopic striae, hyperpigmentation.

F. Rheumatic fever: increased sweating, petechiae, urticaria, erythema marginatum.

G. Ulcerative colitis: spreading pyodermas (pyoderma gangrenosum), ulcers, necrosis.

H. Lipidoses: xanthelasma, or characteristic papules, nodules, plaques of yellowish xanthomas, pruritus.

I. Vitamin deficiencies.
1. Hypovitaminosis A: phrynoderma is dry, hyperkeratotic skin.
2. Hypervitaminosis A: dry skin, exfoliations, hair loss
3. Thiamine (B_1) deficiency: in beriberi there are edematous, erythematous plantar areas.
4. Riboflavin (B_2) deficiency: angular cheilosis, glossitis;
5. Nicotinic acid deficiency: in pellagra fissured, red, exfoliative dermatitis and hyperpigmentation are representative.
6. Ascorbic acid deficiency: in scurvy follicular petechiae, papules, purpura are seen.
7. Vitamin K deficiency: purpura.
8. Vitamin P (hesperidin) deficiency: purpura.

J. Internal carcinomas, lymphomas, leukemias and mycosis fungoides; purpura, pruritus, pyodermas, pigmented (melanin) papillomas and erythematous patches, nodules, excoriations.

K. Neurofibromatosis (von Recklinghausen's disease): patchy melanin hyperpigmentations or cafe-au-lait spots, pedunculated nodules.

TUMORS OF THE SKIN

A. Senile (actinic) keratosis: precancerous lesion, due to sunlight; flat, polygonal, tan-brown colored exfoliative, adherent patches.

Differential diagnosis: seborrheic keratosis, squamous cell carcinoma.

Treatment: (a) electrosurgery; (b) topical dermatologic medications.

B. Cutaneous horn: precancerous lesion, hyperkeratotic, proliferative protuberance.

Differential diagnosis: squamous cell carcinoma.

Treatment: electrosurgery.

C. Leukoplakia: precancerous lesion, whitish flat plaque caused by chronic physical, chemical irritation.

Differential diagnosis: callus, lichen planus.

Treatment: (a) elimination of irritant; (b) electrosurgery; (c) protective dermatologic preparations.

D. Squamous cell carcinoma: rapidly enlarging nodule developing a central ulcer and indurated rolled border with erythema. Keratotic, crusted or verrucous forms can occur.

Differential diagnosis: senile keratosis, basal cell epithelioma.

Treatment: (a) surgery; (b) radiation therapy.

E. Basal cell epithelioma: slowly enlarging nodule with central depression, ulceration, pigmentation, or scarry plaque character.

Differential diagnosis: squamous cell carcinoma, sebaceous adenoma, large acne, verruca, scarring, psoriasis, seborrheic dermatitis.

Treatment: (a) surgical excision; (b) electrocautery.

F. Malignant melanoma: may arise per se or develop from a nevus as a flat, usually nonhairy, brown, spreading pigmentation becoming indurated, elevated, papillomatous or pedunculated, forming an ulcer, bleeding and crusting.

Differential diagnosis: basal cell epithelioma, squamous cell carcinoma, verruca, pedunculated fibroma, granuloma pyogenicum, seborrheic keratosis, lentigo (this is to be differentiated from freckles or ephelides).

Treatment: surgical excision.

G. Mycosis (lymphoma) fungoides: begins as erythematous patches (erythematous stage), with exfoliation, pruritus, developing induration, red, scaly plaques (plaque stage) with central atrophy, and final nodular form (tumor stage) with excoriation and ulceration.

Differential diagnosis: atopic eczema, psoriasis, exfoliative dermatitis, syphilis, erythema multiforme, fungal infections, lymphomas, tuberculosis, leprosy, sarcoidosis.

Treatment: (a) corticosteroids; (b) radiation therapy; (c) systemic medications for lymphomas.

H. Benign neoplasms.

    1. Seborrheic keratosis: small brownish, greasy, warty plaques (slow enlargement).

Differential diagnosis: malignant melanoma, wart, nevus, actinic keratosis.

Treatment: curettement.

    2. Epidermal cyst and sebaceous cyst; 99.5% of a clinical "sebaceous cyst" turns out to be an epidermal cyst during histopathologic examination.

Differenial diagnosis: lipoma, dermoid cyst, mucous retention cyst, synovial cyst.

Treatment: removal of the intact cyst capsule with the cyst content.

    3. Hemangiomas: considered to be hamartomatous vascular abnormalities. Some typical hemangiomas are:

       a. Port-wine stain: diffuse, violaceous patch.

       b. Capillary (senile) hemangioma: small red, flat or elevated tumor.

       c. "Strawberry" tumor: superficial hemangioma and cavernous hemangioma. Are bright red, elevated tumors, start small, may develop large sizes.

       d. Spider hemangioma: central red arteriole with radiating small blood vessels.

Treatment of b. and d. is electrosurgery, c. is cryosurgery.

Cranial Nerve Examination

The function of cranial nerves: afferent or "enter," efferent or "exit."

A. Somatic nerves supply the skin, striated muscles and organs of special sense.

B. Visceral nerves supply the visceral regions and smooth muscles. Both can be special (supply of special functions) or general, e.g., general visceral afferent (visceral sensibility), general somatic afferent (cutaneous sensibility), general visceral efferent (involuntary muscle and gland control), general somatic efferent (tongue movements), special visceral afferent (taste, smell), special somatic afferent (hearing, vision), special visceral efferent (swallowing, phonation), special somatic efferent (head and shoulder movements).

OLFACTORY (I)

Function: smell (special visceral efferent).

Disorder: decreased acuity of smell, dysosmia, anosmia, olfactory hallucinations.

Rule out: herpes simplex, encephalitis, olfactory neuroblastoma (esthesioneuroepithelioma), influenza.

OPTIC (II)

Function: sight (special somatic afferent).

Disorder: impaired visual acuity, scotomas, hemianopia and other visual field defects (central, peripheral), daltonism, amaurosis fugax, visual hallucinations, photophobia.

Rule out: cerebral infarction, cerebral apoplexy, brain abscess, neurosyphilis, intracranial neoplasm, temporal arteritis, diabetic neuropathy, multiple sclerosis.

OCULOMOTOR (III)

Function: motor to orbital muscles (somatic efferent), motor to intraocular muscles (general visceral efferent), general somatic afferent.

Disorder: diplopia, divergent strabismus, ophthalmoplegia due to impaired medial or vertical eye movements, ptosis, mydriatic and fixed pupils (defect of pupillary reaction to light and accommodation), nystagmus, Argyll-Robertson pupil (small irregular, unequal, bilateral; no light reflex seen in neurolues and diabetes mellitus).

Rule out: bulbar poliomyelitis, herpes zoster, neurosyphilis, peripheral oculomotor neuropathy, Wernicke-Korsakoff syndrome, multiple sclerosis, intracranial neoplasm, myasthenia gravis, diabetic neuropathy.

TROCHLEAR (IV)

Function motor to superior oblique (somatic efferent), general somatic afferent.

Disorder: diplopia in downward medial ocular movement.

Rule out: cavernous sinus thrombosis, intracranial infection, neoplasm.

TRIGEMINAL (V)

Function: general somatic afferent, special visceral efferent.

Ophthalmic nerve: sensory perception from frontal, nasal and upper palpebral integument, bulbar and upper palpebral conjunctivae, caruncula lacrimalis, frontal, ethmoidal, sphenoidal sinuses, mucous membrane of the nasal cavity, lacrimal sac and gland (secretory from facial nerve).

Maxillary nerve: sensory impulses from the skin of the middle portion of the face, upper lip, side of the nose, conjunctiva of the lower eyelid, septum mobile nasi, mucous membrane of the upper lip, ethmoidal, sphenoidal and maxillary sinuses, the hard and soft palate, uvula, palatine tonsil, nasopharynx, superior, middle and inferior conchae, nasal septum, mucosa of maxillary tuberosity, adjacent buccal mucosa, upper gingivae, the teeth, alveolar areas, and secretory to the minor salivary glands of these regions through the greater superficial petrosal branch of the facial nerve.

Mandibular nerve: sensory fibers from the skin of the lower part of the face, cheek, lower lip, buccal area, auricala (tragus and helix), external acoustic meatus, tympanic membrane, mastoid air cells, temporal region, temporomandibular joint, buccal mucous membrane, lower gingivae, the teeth, alveolar areas, floor of the mouth, anterior two-thirds of the tongue (chorda tympani conveys impulses of taste, i.e., special visceral afferent of the anterior two-thirds of the tongue), submandibular, sublingual and minor salivary glands (secretory through the chorda tympani of facial nerve, i.e., general visceral efferent); motor supply to the tensores tympani and veli palatini, anterior belly of the digastrici, the mylohyoideus, and the muscles of mastication (the temporalis, the masseter, the pterygoidei).

Disorder: paresthesia, anesthesia, hyperesthesia, pain, altered sensation of face, nose, eyes, oral cavity, or effect on the mandibular movement, deglutition, hearing, sneeze reflex.

Rule out: trigeminal neuralgia, neoplasm of Gasserian ganglion (semilunar), sphenopalatine neuralgia, paratrigeminal syndrome, lingual neoplasm, orolingual paresthesia, herpes zoster.

ABDUCENS (VI)

Function: motor to the lateral rectus muscle (somatic efferent), general somatic afferent.

Disorder: convergent strabismus due to impaired lateral ocular movement.

Rule out: aneurysm of internal carotid artery, increased intracranial pressure.

FACIAL (VII)

Function: motor to the platysma myoid, posterior belly of the digastrici, the stylohyoid, the stapedius and the muscles of the external ear, the occipitalis, the frontalis, the orbicularis oculi, the zygoma, the buccinator, the nose area, the orbicularis oris and the rest of the muscles of facial expression, i.e., special visceral efferent; the chorda tympani conveys taste perception from the anterior two-thirds of the tongue, i.e., special visceral afferent, and supplies secretory impulses to the submandibular and sublingual salivary glands, i.e., general visceral efferent.

Disorder: altered facial expression, spasm, paralysis, asymmetry, eye closure, forehead wrinkle, nasolabial fold, tearing, salivation, and taste sensation of the anterior two-thirds of the tongue.

Rule out: facial paralysis, blepharospasm (involvement of orbicularis), spasmus nictitans (spasm of facial muscles), brain hemorrhage, neoplasm, abscess, middle ear lesions, cranial fractures (base of the skull), parotid involvement, herpes zoster.

ACOUSTIC (VIII)

Function: hearing through the chochlear nerve, and equilibrium by the vestibular nerve, i.e., special somatic afferent.

Disorder: hearing (tinnitus, total or partial deafness due to sensorineural losses), equilibration (dizziness, nausea, gait, vertigo, nystagmus).

Rule out: conductive hearing losses, hereditary deafness, fracture related traumatic hearing loss, middle ear infections, Meniere's disease, neurotropic infections (rubella, syphilis), otosclerosis, multiple sclerosis, neoplasm, seizure, syncope.

GLOSSOPHARYNGEAL (IX)

Function: taste perception of the posterior third and posterior half of the sides of the tongue, i.e., special visceral afferent; sensory to these areas and palatine tonsils, palatine arches, soft palate, the upper and middle part of the pharynx, osseous part of the auditory tube, mastoid cells, tympanic cavity, mucosa of the tympanic membrane, i.e., general visceral afferent; motor to the stylopharyngeus, i.e., special visceral efferent, and secretory for the parotid gland through the lesser superficial petrosal nerve, i.e., general visceral efferent.

Disorder: taste perception of the posterior third of the tongue, altered gag reflex, parotid secretion, dysphagia, neuralgia.

Rule out: glossopharyngeal neuralgia, otitis media, mastoiditis, pharyngitis, lingual tonsilitis, neoplasm.

VAGUS (X)

Function: sensory from the integument of the dorsal part of the auricle, the posteroinferior surface of the external acoustic meatus, i.e., general somatic afferent; general visceral afferent from the lower portion of the pharynx, the base of the tongue, esophagus, internal and pharyngeal surfaces of the larynx, the trachea, the thoracic and abdominal viscera; taste perception of epiglottis region, i.e., special visceral afferent; motor to the lower constrictor muscles of the pharynx, soft palate (except the tensor veli palatini) related to deglutition, the larynx muscles providing phonation, i.e., special visceral efferent; and general visceral efferent to the heart, smooth muscles and glands of the trachea, bronchi, esophagus, stomach and other thoracic and abdominal viscera.

Disorder: dysphagia, regurgitation of fluid and food, vomiting, asymmetric movement (deviation) of the soft palate, speech problems, hoarseness, laryngeal paralysis, aphonia, localized dysgeusia, ageusia, abnormal cardiac and respiratory rate (in vagotomy or pressure of a tumor the pulse is weak, inspiratory dyspnea), bradypnea, asthma, pneumonia, (stridulous breathing, cough, etc.), vasomotor apparatus (vasovagal syncope), functional changes in the abdominal viscera (gastric hyperacidity, peptic ulcer, dysuria, constipation, or postvagotomy diarrhea).

Rule out: injury of the vagus in accidental or surgery wound (common in thyroidectomy, fracture of the base of the skull), pressure of a neoplasm or vacular aneurysm along the course of the vagus, parasympathetic overtone.

ACCESSORY (XI)

Function: motor to the sternocleidomastoid and the trapezius (and by the vagus to the muscles of pharynx and larynx), i.e., special somatic (visceral) efferent; general visceral efferent as integral part of the vagus by the internal ramus.

Disorder: spasm, asthenia or paralysis of sternocleidomastoid, trapezius muscles, altered head position.

Rule out: injury, neoplasm, abscess, disruption of the accessory nerve.

HYPOGLOSSAL (XII)

Function: motor to the thyroid, sternothyroid, omohyoid, hypoglossus, styloglossus, geniohyoideus (innervation from the cervical plexus), genioglossus and the intrinsic striated muscles of the tongue, i.e., general somatic efferent.

Disorder: deviation of the tongue to the affected side on protrusion, lingual tremor, fibrillation, fasciculation, muscular atrophy, hypertrophy.

Rule out: bulbar disease, injured nerve in surgery or accidental wound in the region of lingual triangle, sublingual abscess, pathologic problems of the submandibular salivary glands.

Cranial Nerve Disorders of Dental Interest

A. TRIGEMINAL NEURALGIA

Etiology: multiple sclerosis, Gasserian ganglion tumor, brainstem infarct, circulatory insufficiency of the Gasserian ganglion elicited by reflex vasoconstriction or vasoconstrictor drugs, or usually unidentifiable structural pathology of the central nervous system (idiopathic trigeminal neuralgia).

Clinical manifestations: the pain—often precipitated by touching a trigger zone of the trigeminal area, or routine oral hygiene procedures, mastication, speech—is paroxysmal, short, excessive stabbing spikes, or clustered lancinating, or continuous in character. Spasmodic contractions of the facial muscles or "tic" may or may not accompany the pain. Spontaneous remissions and exacerbations. Generally unilateral.

Differential diagnosis: nasopharyngeal neoplasm, trigeminal neuritis (due to intracranial aneurysm, head neoplasm, dental pathology), migraine, sinusitis, postherpetic (herpes zoster) neuralgia, mechanical trauma of the head and Trotter syndrome (intracranial invasion of neoplasm via foramen ovale, impaired mobility of the soft palate on the tumor side, trismus and neuralgic pain), paratrigeminal syndrome (pain and cephalalgia located in the trigeminal region, miosis due to paralysis of thoracolumbar sympathetic nerve supplying the dilator pupillae).

Treatment: (a) carbamazepine; (b) diphenylhydantoin; (c) neurectomy by surgery or other means.

B. FACIAL PARALYSIS (BELL'S PALSY)

Etiology: accidental trauma, surgical procedures at the area of the parotid gland, caloric changes, e.g., cold air ("trucker's disease"), ischemia of the facial nerve at stylomastoid foramen, internal anditory meatus, herpes zoster of the geniculate ganglion, infections and neoplasms of the cerebellopontine angle and meninges.

Clinical manifestations: sudden onset of unilateral weakness or paralysis of the muscles of facial expression, impaired closure of the eye, drooping and retraction of the angle of the mouth, smooth forehead, cannot raise the eyebrow or wink the eye, dysgeusia of the half of the anterior two-thirds of the tongue, hyperacusis due to paralysis of stapedius muscle, difficulty in masticating, food collects at vestibular sulcus, impaired speech, drooling of saliva from the corner of the mouth and tearing on the affected side.

Prognosis may promise gradual recovery, may be accompanied by spasms of the facial musculature.

Differential diagnosis: chronic facial hemispasm (caused by degeneration of the facial nucleus in the pons), cerebral apoplexy, Melkersson-Rosenthal syndrome (fissured tongue, paroxysmal facial paralysis, cheilitis granuloma, facial edema).

Treatment: (a) corticosteroids; (b) neurosurgery; (c) nicotinic acid, histamine (vasodilators).

C. SPHENOPALATINE NEURALGIA (HORTON'S SYNDROME)

Etiology: ischemia of the sphenopalatine ganglion, sphenoid sinus infection, tumor.

Clinical manifestations: paroxysmal attacks of intense unilateral pain in the region of the ear, eye, nose and face accompanied by nasal discharge, sneezing, tearing and paresthesia of the integument of the affected areas ("periodic migrainous neuralgia"). "Trigger zone" is absent.

Differential diagnosis: Meniere's disease.

Treatment: (a) ergotamine; (b) methysergide; (c) neurosurgery, cautery of the sphenopalatine ganglion.

D. GLOSSOPHARYNGEAL NEURALGIA

Etiology: ischemia of glossopharyngeal nerve, neoplasm, infection.

Clinical manifestations: unilateral, paroxysmal attacks of pain of various intensity located in the posterior third of the tongue, pharynx, palatine tonsil and ear. There is a "trigger zone" somewhere in these locations.

Differential diagnosis: pathologic conditions of the areas involved.

Treatment: neurectomy.

E. MIGRAINE SYNDROME

Etiology: neurogenic or neurohumoral vasoconstriction followed by vasodilatation of the cerebral arteries.

Clinical manifestations: irritability, vertigo, confusion, nausea, diarrhea or constipation, visual hallucinations, scotomas (preheadache phenomenon), culminating in excruciating, deep cephalalgia, vomiting, head and neck muscle contractions, erythema of the conjunctiva, excessive lacrimation. The attacks vary in duration and extent.

Differential diagnosis: sphenopalatine neuralgia, temporal arteritis, cluster or histamine headache, trigeminal neuralgia.

Treatment: (a) ergotamine; (b) propranolol; (c) corticosteroids; (d) methysergide; (e) analgesics.

F. MENIERE'S DISEASE

Etiology: excess pressure of endolymph in the membranous labyrinth caused by dysfunction of vasomotor apparatus in autonomic nervous system disorder, allergic reaction.

Clinical manifestations: persistent unilateral tinnitus, deafness and vertigo, dizziness.

Differential diagnosis: acute and recurrent peripheral vestibulopathy, cardiovascular disease, hypothyroidism, otitis media, cerebral arteriosclerosis.

Treatment: (a) histamine, nicotinic acid (vasodilators); (b) labyrinthotomy; (c) neurectomy of the acoustic nerve.

G. OROLINGUAL PARESTHESIA

Etiology: systemic disorders (diabetic neuropathy, hypogonadism, vitamin and nutritional deficiency, hypothyroidism, megaloblastic anemia, allergy, drug side effect, psychogenic), local (dental, oral habits, tonsillitis, electrogalvanic potential difference between various restorative metals moistened by saliva, infections).

Clinical manifestations: paresthetic burning pain of the oral mucosa, often the tongue (glossopyrosis, glossodynia).

Differential diagnosis: rule out systemic and local disorders such as trigeminal neuralgia, myofascial pain-dysfunction syndrome, depression, referred pain.

Treatment: (a) antidepressants, muscle relaxants; (b) sex hormones; (c) analgesics, topical anesthetics; (d) antibiotics; (e) antihistamines, (f) vitamins.

Head and Neck Lymph Node Examination

In case of lymphadenopathy the inspection of the size of lymph node enlargement is followed by palpation of the lymph nodes for exact location, size and consistency (soft, fluctuant, semihard, stonyhard), movability (freely movable, discrete, fixed, matted), tenderness (nontender, painful). It is generally accepted that normal, healthy lymph nodes are not palpable.

To facilitate the clinical examination of head and neck lymph nodes the next few pages are included to illustrate the topography and drainage areas of the head and neck lymphatic system.

A. LYMPHATIC TRUNKS

Figure 2.26 illustrates the lymphatic trunks.

B. ARRANGEMENT OF HEAD AND NECK LYMPH NODES

It is customary to identify the location of the individual lymph nodes by name, but note that the names denote individually encapsulated lymph nodes being always multiple.

1. The circular arrangement (located at the junction of the head and neck) *and facial lymph nodes* are illustrated in Figure 2.27.

   a. *Circular*

      Occipital: at the attachment of the trapezius muscle (Figure 2.28).

      Posterior auricular: at the insertion of the sternocleidomastoid muscle.

      Anterior auricular: immediately anterior to the tragus.

      Parotid nodes: embedded in the substance of the parotid salivary gland, and located under it on the lateral pharyngeal wall.

      Submandibular: on or in the submandibular salivary gland (tilt the head to the side of the palpation and slightly forward) (Figure 2.29).

      Stahr's: anterior to the external maxillary artery at the base of the mandible.

      Submental (suprahyoid): between the anterior bellies of diagastric muscles (Figure 2.30)

      Lingual: on the hyoglossus muscle and under the genioglossus muscle.

   b. *Facial*

      Epitrochlear: over the trochlea.

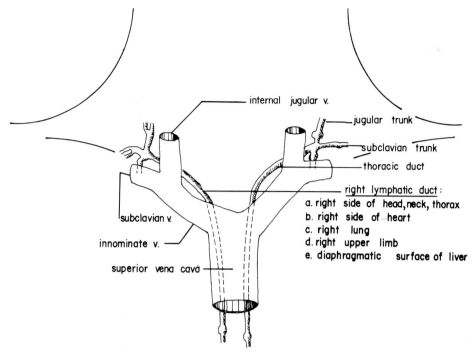

Figure 2.26 Lymphatic trunks.

internal jugular v.

jugular trunk

subclavian trunk

thoracic duct

right lymphatic duct:
a. right side of head, neck, thorax
b. right side of heart
c. right lung
d. right upper limb
e. diaphragmatic surface of liver

subclavian v.

innominate v.

superior vena cava

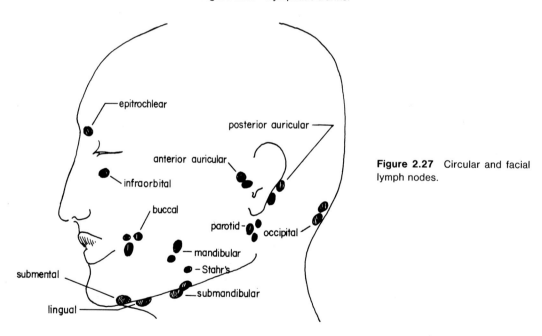

Figure 2.27 Circular and facial lymph nodes.

epitrochlear

posterior auricular

anterior auricular

infraorbital

buccal

parotid

occipital

mandibular

Stahr's

submandibular

submental

lingual

Infraorbital: at infraorbital foramen.
Buccal: over the buccinator muscle.
Mandibular: anterior to the masseter muscle.
Deep facial: between the ramus of the mandible and the lateral pterygoid muscle.

Retropharyngeal: behind the epipharynx on the buccopharyngeal fascia and prevertebral fascia.

2. The cervical arrangement is shown in Figure 2.31.

Tonsillar (subdigastric): this uppermost cervical lymph node is located at the upper

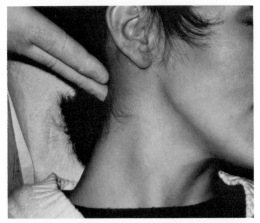

Figure 2.28 Palpation of the occipital lymph nodes.

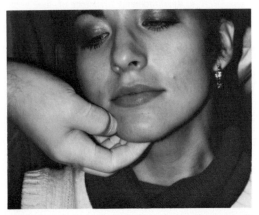

Figure 2.29 Palpation of the submandibular lymph nodes.

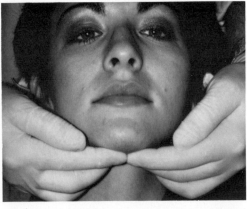

Figure 2.30 Palpation of the submental lymph nodes.

one-third of the posterior belly of the digastric muscle (Figure 2.32).

Superior deep cervical (jugulodigastric): at the crossing point of the internal jugular vein and the posterior (superior) belly of digastric muscle (Figure 2.33).

Principal node of the tongue: at the carotid bifurcation.

Inferior deep cervical (juguloomohyoid): extend beyond the posterior margin of the sternocleidomastoid muscle into the supraclavicular triangle, where they are closely related to the brachial nerve plexus and the subclavian vein. The most inferior portion of them is also called the supraclavicular node (Virchow's is the left supraclavicular lymph node group) (Figures 2.34 and 2.35).

Superficial cervical: located in close relationship with the external jugular vein and superficial to the sternocleidomastoid muscle (Figure 2.36).

Posterior cervical: over the scalene muscles (Figure 2.37).

DRAINAGE

Scalp: parotid, anterior auricular, posterior auricular and occipital and inferior deep cervical.

Face: submental, submandibular, parotid and superior deep cervical.

Nasal cavity: submandibular, retropharyngeal and superior deep cervical.

Oral cavity: as illustrated in Figure 2.38.

Common Primary and Secondary Lymphadenopathies of the Head and Neck Areas

A. MALIGNANT LYMPHOMA

1. *Giant Follicular Hyperplasia*

Clinical manifestations: insidious onset, slow progress, discrete, painless, soft enlargement of superficial lymph nodes, splenomegaly.

2. *Hodgkin's Disease*

Clinical manifestations: Pel-Ebstein's fever is characterized by alternating periods (3 to 10 days) of febrile and afebrile cycles. Malaise, anorexia, weight loss; anemia (easy bruising, hemorrhages, dyspnea, cephalalgia, tinnitus, asthenia, palpitations, tachycardia, pallor); night sweats, severe, generalized pruritus; development of "mycosis fungoides"; dysphagia; persistent, painless, rubbery-firm enlargement of lymph nodes covered by normal skin; peripheral neuritis and pain due to the tumor growth, the pressure of enlarged lymph

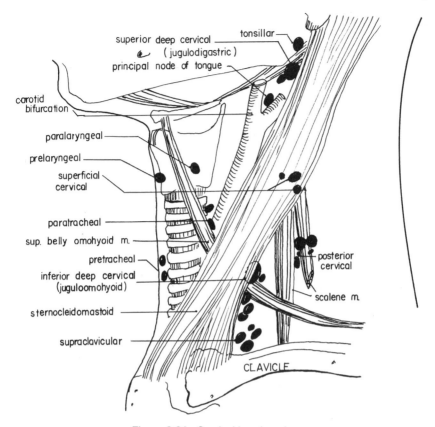

Figure 2.31 Cervical lymph nodes.

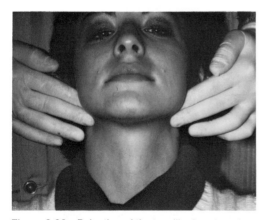

Figure 2.32 Palpation of the tonsillar lymph nodes.

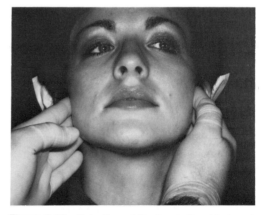

Figure 2.33 Palpation of the jugulodigastric lymph nodes.

nodes, and in the region of lymph node involvement following alcohol intake.

Treatment: (a) radiotherapy; (b) chemotherapy—vinblastine, vincristine (Oncovin), cyclophosphamide, nitrogen mustard, procarbazine and chlorambucil; (c) combination chemotherapy—MOPP program (nitrogen mustard, oncovin, procar-

bazine and prednisone); (d) combined radiotherapy and chemotherapy.

3. Reticulum Cell Sarcoma and Lymphosarcoma

Clinical manifestations: rubbery, hard, fixed, early painless and late painful lymph node enlargement covered by red-

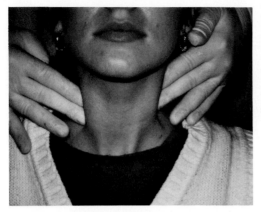

Figure 2.34 Palpation of the juguloomohyoid lymph nodes.

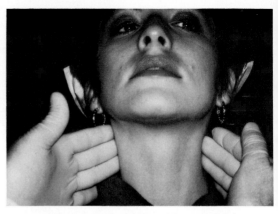

Figure 2.36 Bilateral palpation of the superficial cervical lymph nodes.

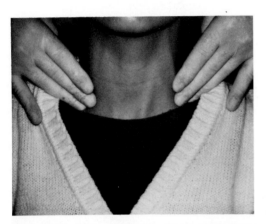

Figure 2.35 Bilateral palpation of the supraclavicular lymph nodes.

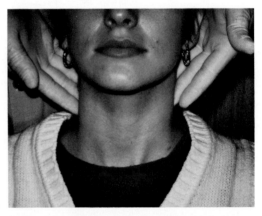

Figure 2.37 Bilateral palpation of the posterior cervical lymph nodes.

dened brawny integument. Naso-oropharynx, tonsils and the rest of the gastrointestinal tract are frequent sites of involvement, causing epistaxis, obstruction, sore throat and hemorrhages. Rapid growth, necrosis and ulcer development are characteristic.

Treatment: (a) radiation therapy; (b) in case of primary reticulum cell sarcoma of bone the radical surgical excision is considered.

4. Acute Leukemias

Clinical manifestations: often generalized lymphadenopathy, hepatosplenomegaly; generalized gingival hyperplasia; anemia (pallor, asthenia, dyspnea, edema, etc.); hemorrhagic manifestations; "leukemic fever"; intercurrent infections.

Treatment: (a) chemotherapy—vincristine, prednisone, 6-mercaptopurine, methotrexate, cytosine arabinoside, and Daunorubicin; (b) radiation treatment in central nervous system leukemia; (c) immunotherapy.

5. Chronic Lymphocytic Leukemia

Clinical manifestations: low grade fever, night sweats; malaise, anorexia, fatigue; enlarged, painful lymph nodes, splenomegaly; intense pruritus, papular, vesicular lesions, herpes zoster; hemorrhagic manifestations.

Treatment: (a) chemotherapeutic agents; (b) chlorambucil.

6. Malignant Neoplasms with Lymph Node Metastasis.
e.g., carcinoma, lymphoepithelioma presenting swelling of the regional lymph nodes.

7. Tuberculosis

Clinical manifestations: The lymphohematogenous dissemination, such as tuber-

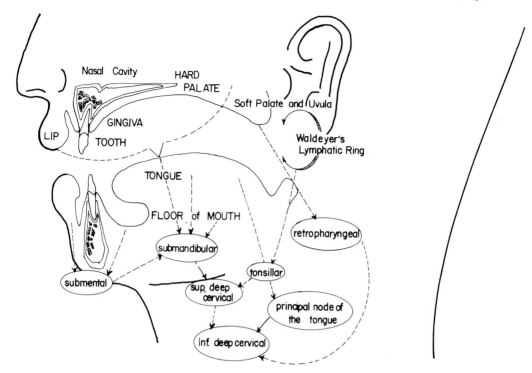

Figure 2.38   Lymphatic drainage of the oral area.

culous lymphadenitis, and the intracana-
licular spread, or direct contact invasion
from pulmonary tuberculosis most frequently present as superficial lymph node
involvement at cervical (tuberculous cervical lymphadenitis or scrofula) and mediastinal regional nodes. These nodes are
usually painless or, less frequently, tender,
painful, form a "cold" abscess, become
fluctuant, show inflammation and perforation of the overlying skin, forming draining fistula by discharging pus.

Treatment: (a) antituberculotic medications—isoniazid, rifampin, streptomycin,
ethambutol, para-aminosalicylic acid, pyr-
izinamide and capreomycin; (b) surgical
resection of draining nodes.

8. Syphilis

Clinical manifestations: The regional
lymph node is always enlarged, draining
the area of the chancre presenting as nonsuppurating, freely movable, firm, painless
"bubovenereal" (buboindolent). In the secondary stage generalized superficial
lymphadenitis is characteristic, involving
the epitrochlear, occipital, post- and
preauricular lymph nodes that are firm,
painless and freely movable.

Treatment: *antibiotics*—penicillin,
erythromycin, tetracycline.

9. Mycotic Infections and Actinomy-
cosis. Paracoccidioidomycosis, cryptococ-
cosis, histoplasmosis, sporotrichosis and
coccidioidomycosis are prone to develop
regional or generalized lymphadenopathy;
first, freely movable nodules become attached to the skin, ulcerate and drain pus.

Treatment: (a) antimycotics—amphotericin B and nystatin; (b) surgical excision;
(c) antibiotics for the actinomycosis—penicillin, tetracycline.

10. Viral Infections. Primary herpes
simplex stomatitis, acute lymphonodular
pharyngitis, herpangina, hand, foot and
mouth disease cause tender regional
lymphadenopathy, as seen in benign lym-
phoreticulosis (cat-scratch disease) with
additional necrosis, suppuration, perforation and discharge. In infectious mononucleosis and acute viral hepatitis generalized lymph node hyperplasia is present
mainly at the cervical, axillary, inguinal
and mediastinal regions. Nodes are slightly
tender, firm, nonsuppurating, freely movable. In addition there may be tender hepatomegaly, splenomegaly, pharyngitis,

fever, nausea, vomiting, hemorrhagic manifestations.

Treatment: no effective specific therapy is available; fortunately, the viral infections are self-limiting.

11. Systemic Lupus Erythematosus

Clinical manifestations: enlarged, nontender, discrete lymph nodes; arthralgias, muscle pain; fever, fatigue, anorexia, nausea, vomiting; "butterfly rash;" hematuria, pyuria, edema; chest pain (pleuritic); anxiety, depression, paranoid reactions.

Treatment: (a) corticosteroids; (b) immunosuppressives; (c) salicylates; (d) antimalarials.

12. Oral, dental infections, like pericoronitis, acute necrotizing ulcerative gingivitis, advanced suppurative periodontitis, periodontal abscess, periapical abscess, osteomyelitis, periostitis, necrotizing ulcerations of the oral mucous membrane can cause tender, localized regional lymphadenopathy.

Treatment: (a) antibiotics; (b) removal of the focus of infection; (c) supportive, symptomatic measures.

Thyroid Gland and Laryngeal Complex

The location of the thyroid gland is shown in Figure 2.39. Palpation of the thyroid gland is illustrated in Figure 2.40. The best accepted technique to palpate the thyroid gland is to approach the neck of the patient in a sitting position from behind, displace the trachea laterally about 1 cm with the fingers of one hand and palpate under the anterior margin of the sternocleidomastoid muscle with the fingers of the other hand during deglutition. Note any nodular or diffuse enlargement, consistency, tenderness and location.

To examine the laryngeal complex displace slightly the thyroid cartilage to both the left and right repeatedly to detect crepitus; record the presence or absence of movement of the laryngeal prominence during deglutition and the position of the trachea at the location of the jugular notch. Deviation of the trachea constitutes an important sign of either atelectasis (toward the affected side) or pleural effusion (away from the involved side). Absence of the crepitus, fixation of the larynx and deviation of the trachea from the midline are warning signs and may signify an inflammatory process or neoplasm.

Disorders of the Thyroid Gland

A. HYPERTHYROIDISM AND GRAVES' DISEASE

Clinical manifestations: goiter, symmetrical or lobulated, firm; exophthalmos, proptosis; tremor, restlessness, insomnia, tachycardia; fatigue, weight loss, cold tolerance, heat intolerance, dyspnea, palpitations, pruritus, reduced visual acuity, abdominal pain; generalized (usually nontender) lymphadenopathy; quick responses, anxiety, hyperreflexia; characteristic fine

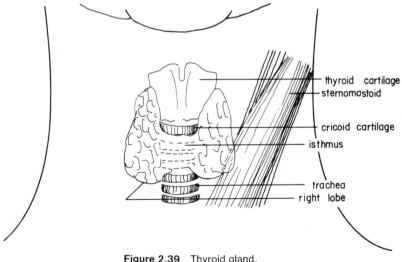

Figure 2.39   Thyroid gland.

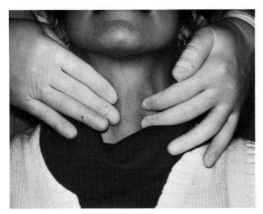

Figure 2.40   Palpation of the thyroid gland.

skin and appendages, excess perspiration, ankle edema.

Treatment: (a) antithyroid medications—propylthiouracil and methimazole; (b) subtotal thyroidectomy.

B. HASHIMOTO'S THYROIDITIS

Clinical manifestations: diffuse thyroid enlargement, soft, may be lobulated, tender; symptoms of hypothyroidism; dysphagia, choking sensation may be present.

Treatment: thyroid hormone therapy.

C. ACUTE AND SUBACUTE THYROIDITIS

Clinical manifestations: partial or total nodular enlargement of the thyroid gland, covered by erythematous intact integument; thyroid area tender to palpation, bilateral radiating pain in the thyroid, mandible and ears, dysphagia, pressure sensation in the neck; fever, pharyngitis, fatigue.

Treatment: (a) analgesia; (b) desiccated thyroid; (c) corticosteroids.

D. HYPOTHYROIDISM AND MYXEDEMA

Clinical manifestations: the thyroid gland may be enlarged, e.g., in the final stage of Hashimoto's thyroiditis, severe iodine deficiency, hypopituitarism; sluggishness, somnolence, cold intolerance; hyporeflexia, edema, coarse dry skin, thick hair, lack of perspiration, joint pain and stiffness; "myxedema madness," frank paranoia, overt psychosis.

Treatment: (a) desiccated thyroid; (b) liotrix (mixture of T3, T4).

E. MULTINODULAR GOITER

Clinical manifestations: asymmetric, progressive enlargement of the thyroid gland, nodularity by palpation; feeling of asphyxia, tracheal compression, hoarseness, cough.

Treatment: (a) desiccated thyroid; (b) surgical resection.

F. TOXIC NODULAR GOITER

Clinical manifestations: multinodular thyroid enlargement; hyperthyroidism (thyrotoxicosis).

Treatment: (a) antithyroid drugs; (b) thyroidectomy.

G. ENDEMIC GOITER

Clinical manifestations: nodular or diffuse bilateral thyroid enlargement; dyspnea, dysphagia.

Treatment: (a) iodine; (b) thyroidectomy.

H. THYROID ADENOMA

Clinical manifestations: presence of a single, painless or sometimes tender nodule; dysphagia, hoarseness.

Treatment: (a) subtotal lobectomy, resection of the nodules; (b) permanent thyroid hormone replacement therapy.

I. THYROID CANCER

Clinical manifestations: early cervical lymph node metastasis, local invasion in the neck; uni- or multicentric nodular masses.

Treatment: (a) surgery (subtotal or total thyroidectomy, radical block dissection and resection of the regional lymph nodes); (b) chemotherapy; (c) thyroid hormone replacement.

Nose

Evaluate for olfactory nerve involvement and the sense of smell. Observe patency or obturation, deviation of the anterior portion of the nasal septum, movement of the alae of the nose (distension during inspiration is often seen in patients with respiratory disease or in extreme distress), anterior nasal discharge, the amount and character (color, odor), enlargement (hammer nose or rhinophyma, myxedema, acromegaly), saddle nose (tertiary syphilis, injury), stuffiness, coryza, sneezing, epistaxis (amount, frequency, duration), palpate for injuries or fractures, tenderness, use rhinoscopy, if indicated, to see the deviation of the nasal septum, inflammatory edema of the nasal mucosa, location of the hemorrhage or foreign material, status of choanae, conchae, and hiatus semilunaris (in case of pain over the maxillary sinus).

Obliteration of nasal air passages prevents endodontic therapy (application of a rubber dam), full mouth prosthetic impressions, extensive oral and periodontal surgeries, the use of water spray for the high-speed dental preparations, nitrous oxide analgesia, etc.

In case of influenza, common cold and other upper respiratory tract infections, the dental treatment is contraindicated to prevent the direct transmission of these diseases to the dental personnel. Furthermore, in patients suffering pulmonary (bronchial) asthma, dental treatment may promote serious respiratory failure.

Dental and nasal infections need to be differentiated from acute and chronic maxillary sinusitis: pain, swelling over the sinus, vague tenderness, and a stuffy sensation on the affected side of the face. Pressure over the sinus or sudden lifting of the head elicits a pain sensation in the sinus area. The breath is fetid and purulent discharge into the nasal cavity is characteristic. Malaise, fatigue and slight fever are present. The choice of treatment is antibiotics and/or surgery. Persistent headache, the "sinus" headache, is the problem of chronic suppurative mucosal inflammation of the paranasal air sinuses (maxillary, frontal, ethmoid, sphenoid); the engorgement and inflammation of the turbinates, nasofrontal ducts and superior nasal spaces may result in osteomyelitis of the adjacent cranial tissues. The headache represents dull recurrent pain which can be relieved by analgesics and decongestants. Offensive nasal discharge is seen in severe rhinitis, syphilitic infection, impacted foreign bodies and advanced systemic lupus erythematosus.

Eyes

Observe the *width of pupils*. A wide, dilated pupil is seen in glaucoma, sympathetic overflow, oculomotor paralysis due to brain lesion, atropine administration or the deep stage of general anesthesia. A narrow, contracted pupil is seen in opiate addiction, alcohol intoxication, or the early stage of general anesthesia. If only one pupil is constricted sympathetic paralysis of the homolateral side or contralateral oculomotor initiation is present. Also observe the *equality and roundness of the pupils* (Argyll Robertson pupil = diabetes mellitus, neurosyphilis); *reaction to light and accommodation*; size, puffiness, prominence (exophthalmos, proptosis); *enophthalmos*; *palpebral fissure* (logophthalmos or the eye cannot be completely closed, ptosis or drooping may be a congenital defect or due to paralysis); *periorbital edema* (in renal disease, congestive heart failure); *palpebrae* (encrustations about the eyelid in hypovitaminosis A; hordeolum in iron deficient anemia; xanthelasma in disturbed lipid metabolism), *inability to move the eyebrows* (may indicate palsy); *the state of adnexa*; the *lacrimal glands and ducts* (excessive lacrimation, xerophthalmia); *cornea* (film, opacity, vascularity and the cataract of the lens); *conjunctivae* (bulbar, palpebral, inner and outer canthi, look for inflammation, abnormal burning or itching sensation, site of frank pain); *color appearance* (the conjunctivae are pale in anemia, yellow sclerae in icterus); *vision* (failing at night only or night blindness, the degree, duration and progression of visual failure, blurring, diplopia, photophobia, scotomas, color blindness), *glasses or contact lenses*, *eye movements* (medial, lateral, vertical and diagonal to indicate the functions of the third, fourth, and sixth cranial nerves, nystagmus, convergent or divergent strabismus). *Palpate* for enlarged lacrimal glands (Mikulicz's disease, Gougerat-Sjögren's syndrome).

Temporomandibular Joint

The examination of the status of temporomandibular joints should include the inspection, palpation and percussion of adjacent areas for abnormalities.

EXTERNAL EAR

Examination of the auricle and tragus (tophi or urate deposits found over the cartilage of the external ear are indicative of gout) will reveal injuries, postauricular scar or depression (mastoidectomy), Blainville's congenital asymmetry, size, color.

EXTERNAL AUDITORY MEATUS

Examine for foreign body, cerumen, abrasion or inflammation (external otitis) eliciting pain, ringing or buzzing sensation, discharge (character and amount).

Palpate for swelling, fluctuation, tenderness (the tragus pain indicating acute infection of the external auditory meatus is at a different location than the preauricular pain present in an inflammatory disorder of the mandibular condyle area). Use the simple otoscope, if indicated, to establish the differential diagnosis, by introducing the funnel with care while the pinna is retracted posterosuperiorly and the tragus is probed gently. Record the symptoms related, like tinnitus, vertigo, otalgia (location and character), deafness (right or left, degree). Inspect the limitations of opening and closing movements of the mandible during protrusion, lateral excursion (the mandible is halfway open), opening and closing, the pattern of deviation from the median sagittal plane asymmetry in mandibular motion, hypo- and hypermobility, occlusal movements (Figures 2.41 to 2.46). Palpation is bilateral to detect the condylar rotation, the symmetry of translocation and the degree of lag as perceived at the pretragus region or in the orifice of the external auditory meatus by the insertion of the little finger (Figure 2.47). The muscles of mastication (opening and closing)

and the cervical musculature (Figure 2.48 and 2.49) are evaluated by palpation. Note the presence of crepitus (clicking) or pain over the articular capsule, the tension, tenderness and spasm of the muscles. Auscultation for crepitus offers further clarity.

Disorders of the Temporomandibular Joint

A. TEMPOROMANDIBULAR JOINT PAIN-DYSFUNCTION SYNDROME

Etiology: decreased or overextended vertical dimension of occlusion; bruxism, clenching related muscle fatigue; traumatic occlusion and minor shifting for centric occlusion; psychosomatic aspects (maladjusted marital status, anxiety reaction).

Clinical manifestations: tenderness, pain of masticatory and cervical muscles

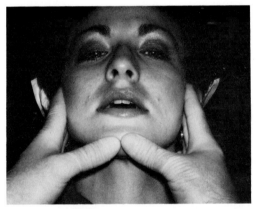

Figure 2.41 Bilateral palpation of the TMJ protrusion.

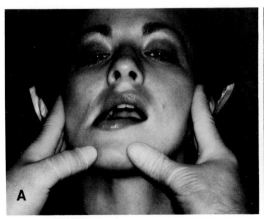

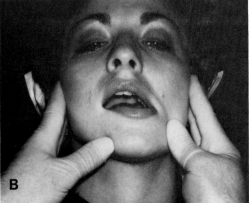

Figure 2.42 *A* and *B*. Bilateral palpation of TMJ during lateral excursion (right and left).

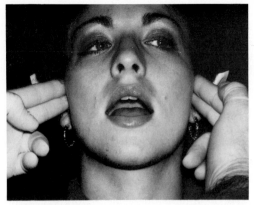

Figure 2.43 Bilateral palpation of TMJ during opening and closing.

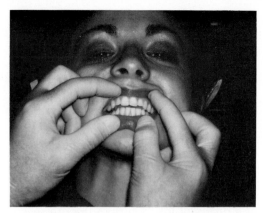

Figure 2.46 Evaluating the cuspid rise.

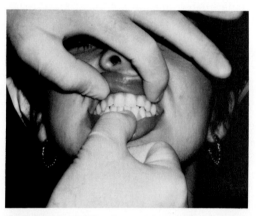

Figure 2.44 Guiding the teeth into the initial centric occlusal contact.

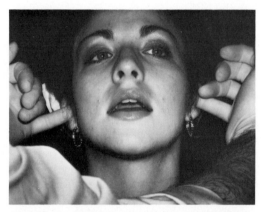

Figure 2.47 Bilateral perception of condyles via external auditory meatus.

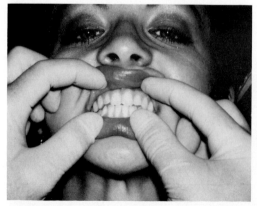

Figure 2.45 Trekking on the incisal guidance.

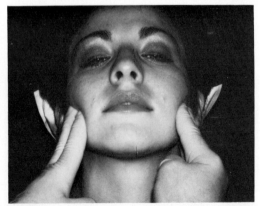

Figure 2.48 Palpation of the masseter muscles.

(uni- or bilateral, spontaneous or upon palpation); crepitus in the temporomandibular joints, but tenderness is absent in the area; limitation of mandibular movements and deviation on opening; infrequently, vertigo, subluxation or habitual dislocation is present.

Treatment: (a) muscle relaxants, tran-

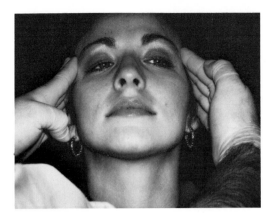

Figure 2.49 Palpation of the temporal muscles.

quilizers, intraarticular steroids; (b) physiotherapy, myotherapy; (c) full mouth rehabilitation; (d) psychotherapy.

B. DEGENERATIVE JOINT DISEASE (OSTEOARTHRITIS)

Clinical manifestations: crepitus with or without pain; impaired mandibular motion.

Treatment: elimination of posterior bite collapse, disturbed occlusal balance or tooth loss.

C. RHEUMATOID ARTHRITIS

Clinical manifestations: swollen, stiff and painful bilateral involvement of the temporomandibular joint with or without crepitus; limited mandibular movements; severe tenderness of the temporomandibular joint area upon palpation; spontaneous remission and exacerbations; slight fever, weight loss, fatigability generally coinciding with acute systemic arthritic episodes; development of joint deformity.

Treatment: (a) intraarticular steroids; (b) antirheumatic medications; (c) condylectomy in ankylosis.

D. LUXATION (AND SUBLUXATION)

Etiology: habitual due to laxity of capsule and ligaments (mouth opened too widely for biting or yawning), traumatic injury (accident, extraction, tonsillectomy).

Clinical manifestations: Subluxation (hypermobility of the condyles extends to the position anterior to the articular emi-

nences) is a habitual problem. The luxation (complete dislocation of the condyles to the front of the articular eminences without spontaneous return to the glenoid fossae) presents locking of the mandible in the open position, painful spasmodic contraction of the temporal, masseter and internal pterygoid muscles. If traumatic luxation is encountered by the impaction of condyles into the posterior-superior bone plate of the glenoid fossae it prevents mandibular movements.

Treatment: (a) reduction of the luxation—manual pressure, central muscle relaxants (Robaxin); (b) reduction of fracture and retention.

E. MENISCUS DISORDERS

Etiology: traumatic injury (acute accidental, extreme mandibular excursion, chronic in malocclusion), specific, nonspecific infections and inflammatory conditions.

Clinical manifestations: dull pain during mandibular motion or at rest position of the mandible, sometimes radiating; crepitus; transient locking of the mandible in central occlusion.

Treatment: (a) bite (night) guard, immobilization; (b) analgesics; (c) correction of malocclusion, posterior bite collapse; (d) meniscectomy.

Salivary Glands and Salivary Flow

A. MAJOR SALIVARY GLANDS

1. Parotid Gland (Figure 2.50). Located in the preauricular area, slightly over the masseter muscle extending behind the posterior border of the mandibular ramus. Inspect the parotid region for any swellings (discrete masses, general enlargement), asymmetry, as well as the area of Stensen's duct opening. Bilateral palpation of the normal parotid glands presents difficulty in distinguishing them from the surrounding tissues. Note any abnormality (pain, tumor) and characteristics present. Bimanual palpation along the course of Stensen's duct, parotid papilla and duct orifice region is followed by drying of the ductal opening and massage ("milking") of the gland: apply firm pressure on the posterior portion of the parotid and carry the

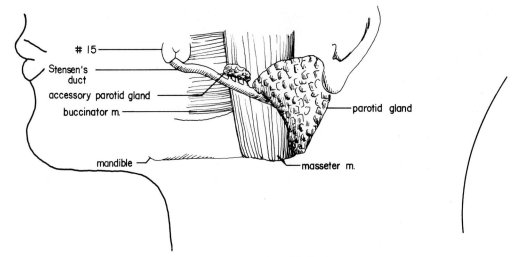

Figure 2.50   Parotid gland.

pressure along the duct. This test allows the dentist to detect ductal obstruction, tenderness (inflammation), and to estimate the degree of salivary flow. The expressed parotid saliva is normally clear, colorless and odorless. The extruded amount is generally a small drop (Figures 2.51 and 2.52).

2. *Submandibular Salivary Gland* (Figure 2.53). Located in the posterior part of the submandibular triangle. The greater part of the gland is superficial, while a small deep portion curves around the posterior free margin of the mylohyoid muscle. The gland is drained by Wharton's duct which arises from the deep portion of the gland and opens just lateral to the lingual frenum at the summit of the sublingual caruncle. Observe any enlargement at the submandibular region in the inferomedial direction. Palpate bilaterally the submandibular glands by exercising superolateral pressure with the fingers while the patient relaxes the tongue. Rule out submandibular lymphadenopathy; the lymph node can be intraglandular (within the submandibular salivary gland). Bimanual palpation is performed (Figures 2.54 and 2.55) by pressing the index finger onto the floor of the mouth while the fingers of the other hand palpate the submandibular salivary gland. Finally, wipe dry the opening of Wharton's duct and apply forward-upward pressure at the posterior portion of the submandibular triangle over the region of the submandibular gland by drawing the fingers anteriorly. Estimate the

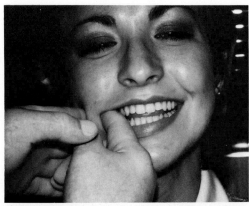

Figure 2.51   Bimanual palpation of Stensen's duct.

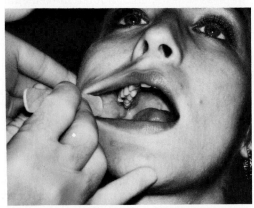

Figure 2.52   Milking the parotid salivary gland to see a bleb of saliva at Stensen's duct orifice.

quality and quantity of usually a small amount of freely flowing, secreted saliva; or in its absence suspect the presence of obliteration of Wharton's duct. Record all

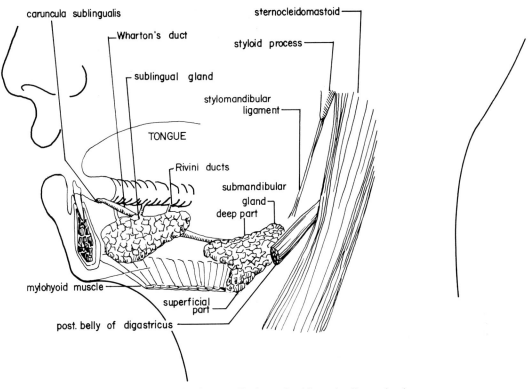

caruncula sublingualis

Wharton's duct

sublingual gland

TONGUE

Rivini ducts

mylohyoid muscle

post. belly of digastricus

superficial part

sternocleidomastoid

styloid process

stylomandibular ligament

submandibular gland

deep part

Figure 2.53 Submandibular and sublingual salivary gland.

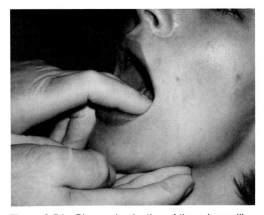

Figure 2.54 Bimanual palpation of the submandibular and sublingual salivary gland.

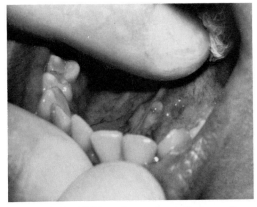

Figure 2.55 Milking the submandibular salivary gland to gain a bleb of saliva from Wharton's duct opening.

the detected abnormalities. If sialadenitis, sialadenosis or sialadenoma, etc. is presumed special diagnostic procedures, such as sequential salivary scintigraphy and sialography are indicated.

3. Sublingual Salivary Gland (Figure 2.53). This gland is found immediately under the mucous membrane of the floor of

the mouth (sublingual fold or plica sublingualis), resting on the mylohyoid muscle. It can be easily inspected and palpated at the middle third of the tongue, close to the attachments of the extrinsic tongue muscles. The duct pattern of the sublingual gland is variable: most of the ducts open along the crest of the plica sublingualis (ducts of Rivinus), while one major duct (Bartholin's) can join to Wharton's duct and open commonly with or along it.

B. MINOR (ACCESSORY) SALIVARY GLANDS

Named after their location: labial, buccal, palatine, inferior apical lingual (Blandin-Nuhn), tonsillar (Weber's) and retromolar (Carmalt's).

Palpate the mucosa to discover any submucosal nodule (rule out sclerosed blood vessels, lymphadenopathy), dry a selected area, e.g., palate or everted lower lip mucosa, and observe the formation of the small droplets of secreted saliva (it takes about 60 seconds to see the droplets) (Figure 2.56).

Disorders of the Salivary Glands

A. SIALOLITHIASIS

Etiology: calcium apatite structure formation in the salivary ducts and ductules with a nidus of microorganisms, cells and breakdown substances.

Clinical manifestations: swelling, pain of the salivary gland; obliteration of the duct lumen can result in the absence of the salivary flow from the duct opening.

Treatment: (a) removal of the small sialolith or the salivary sand by massage of the gland and manipulations along the duct; (b) sialolithotomy.

B. MUMPS (EPIDEMIC PAROTITIS)

Etiology: RNA virus.

Clinical manifestations: usually bilateral, resilient, diffuse, tender swelling of the salivary glands, commonly the parotid; slight fever, cephalalgia, nausea, vomiting.

Treatment: supportive management.

C. MUCOVISCIDOSIS (CYSTIC FIBROSIS)

Etiology: hereditary disorder.

Clinical manifestations: bilateral salivary gland swellings; sialorrhea, excessive sputum production.

Treatment: antibiotics.

D. POSTOPERATIVE SIALADENITIS

Etiology: normal commensals of the oral cavity invading retrograde the glands in

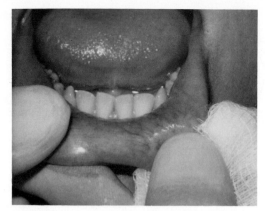

Figure 2.56 Inspection of salivary secretions from labial glands.

dehydrated, xerostomic and debilitated patients (streptococci, staphylococci, etc.)

Clinical manifestations: painful swelling of the salivary gland, purulent discharge through the duct orifice upon manipulation over the gland and duct; moderate fever, trismus, prostration, anorexia.

Treatment: (a) antibiotics; (b) supportive measurements.

E. METABOLIC SALIVARY GLAND HYPERTROPHY

Etiology: malnutrition, diabetes mellitus, chronic alcoholic hepatitis and cirrhosis of the liver.

Clinical manifestations: asymptomatic, diffuse, bilateral, progressive enlargement of the salivary glands; systemic signs and symptoms of the basic metabolic disorder.

Treatment: correction and control of the systemic disorder.

F. SJÖGREN'S SYNDROME

Etiology: autoimmunization is suggested.

Clinical manifestations: swelling of the salivary glands; xerostomia, dysgeusia; rheumatoid arthritis; keratoconjunctivitis sicca, xerophthalmia; buccopharyngolaryngitis sicca; tenderness of the dry areas.

Treatment: (a) corticosteroids; (b) symptomatic.

G. MIKULICZ'S DISEASE

Etiology: autoimmunity is suspected.

Clinical manifestations: enlarged salivary glands; xerostomia, dysgeusia, tenderness; swelling of the lacrimal glands.

Treatment: (a) corticosteroids; (b) surgical excision in the case of formation of a discrete neoplasm.

H. PLEOMORPHIC ADENOMA (MIXED TUMOR)

Clinical manifestations: lobulated, firm neoplasm of various nature (benign, malignant) and sizes. (a) benign—painless, freely movable, slowly forming, covered by normal integument; (b) malignant, fast growing, frequently painful, fixed, surface ulceration, nerve paralysis.
Treatment: surgical excision.

I. ADENOCARCINOMA

Clinical manifestations: early pain, fixed mass, surface ulceration, nerve paralysis.
Treatment: (a) surgery; (b) radiation.

J. MUCOEPIDERMOID CARCINOMA

Clinical manifestations: (a) low-grade malignancy—painless, slow enlargement, cystic areas; (b) high-grade malignancy—painful, nerve paralysis, rapid enlargement, surface ulceration.
Treatment: (a) surgery; (b) radiation.

K. ADENOSQUAMOUS CARCINOMA

Clinical manifestations: small oral ulcer; indurated submucosal nodule; fast growth.
Treatment: (a) surgery; (b) radiation.

L. SQUAMOUS CELL CARCINOMA (EPIDERMOID CARCINOMA)

Clinical manifestations: small submucosal nodule; intraglandular discrete mass in the major salivary gland; fast growth; painless.
Treatment: (a) surgery; (b) radiation.

Lips

Two tongue blades are used to examine the intraoral soft tissues (Figures 2.57 to 2.61). *Observe* the position of the lips at rest (open resting lips indicate mouth breathing), the skin surface, vermilion border, moist mucosa, commissures, frenal attachments, and labial vestibuli, the color, hue (uniform, pink), the general appearance and abnormalities (developmental anomalies, i.e., cleft lip, lip pits); dry, dessiccated (dehydration, circulatory insuffi-

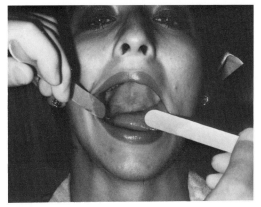

Figure 2.57 Two tongue blades are used for general inspection of the oral cavity.

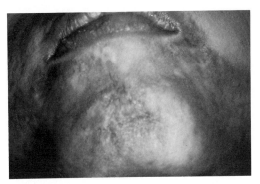

Figure 2.58 Burn (scarring and pigmentation).

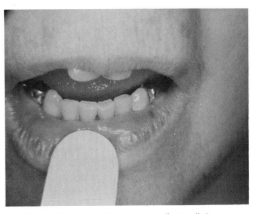

Figure 2.59 Amalgam tattoo (lower lip).

ciency), edematous (angioneurotic edema, Melkersson-Rosenthal syndrome characterized by facial paralysis, fissured tongue and cheilitis granulomatosa; cheilitis granulomatosa, per se); pale, white (anemia), deep red, blotchy (severe systemic arterial hypertension, congestive heart failure, polycythemia), stripped or speckled with

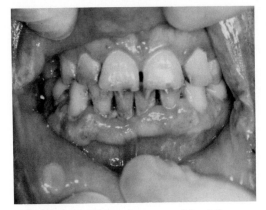

Figure 2.60   2° lues (mucous patches), lip.

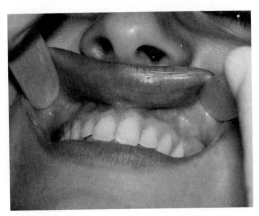

Figure 2.61   Inspection of the upper lip and adjacent areas.

melanotic freckles (Peutz-Jeghers syndrome having intestinal polyps, melanotic freckles of Hutchinson), presence of elementary and specific lesions (abrasion, erosion, necrosis, ulcer, fissure, e.g., cheilitis, syphilitic rhagades, chancre, split papule, maceration, perlèche or angular cheilosis, crusting, laceration, contusion, petechiae, ecchymosis, vibex, vesicles, bullae, e.g., pemphigus, frank hemorrhages (e.g., leukemia) draining, oozing (e.g., epidermoid cyst)). *Palpate* for tenderness, pain (localized or diffuse infection, inflammation), seen or unseen masses (Figure 2.62, a and b); sclerosed submucosal blood vessels, fibrosed minor salivary glands and lymphatic nodules (nonencapsulated) and to detect texture and consistency (spongy, indurated smooth, coarse, irregular, granular, raised masses or swellings, firm filamentuous, e.g., scleroderma), sensory and motor dysfunctions. Observe the minor

salivary gland duct openings and secretory function. In describing the location and characteristics of the detected lesion the use of the anatomical rubber stamps will facilitate the procedure of clinical evaluation and clear understanding.

Include the following: size, shape, location, contour; margins (regular, smooth, irregular, coarse, undetermined or diffuse, sharp or well defined, inflammatory hyperemia, edematous, elevated, indurated, granulating, friable, purulent, hemorrhagic); base (pedunculated, superficial, deep or crateriform, soft, indurated, fibrinous, seropurulent, necrotic, crusted, granulomatous).

Buccal Mucosae and Vestibular Sulci

Inspect the area of Stensen's duct openings, the parotid papillae, degree of moisture of the mucous membrane, the distribution of frenal attachments, obliteration of the mucobuccal folds. *Palpate* by using bimanual technique (one hand is on the

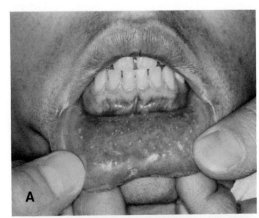

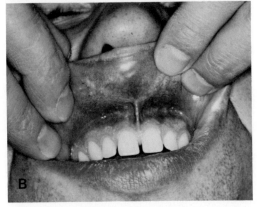

Figure 2.62   *A.* Inspection and palpation of the lower lip region. *B.* Palpation of the upper lip.

skin surface of the cheek area, the other is on the inner cheek). Describe in detail any patches, discoloration or lesion, the area of tenderness, the location and characteristics of the lumps (Figures 2.63 to 2.65).

Disorders Frequently Encountered

A. LEUKOEDEMA

Etiology: unidentified.

Clinical manifestations: opalescent film, may assume coarsely corrugated appearance. Stretching the area results in disappearance of the whitish hue.

Treatment: watchful waiting to identify any transition of this condition to clinical leukoplakia.

B. LEUKOPLAKIA

Etiology: multifactorial, such as systemic influences (avitaminosis A, vitamin B complex deficiency, insufficiency of sex hormones), local chronic irritation of the mucous membranes (concentrated al-

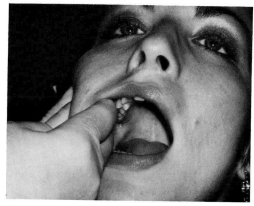

Figure 2.65 Bimanual palpation of the buccal region.

cohol, tobacco smoking or chewing, snuff dipping, heavy supragingival calculosis, sharp protuberant dental restorations, electrogalvanism, "morsicatio buccarum, labiorum"), candida albicans infection ("speckled" leukoplakia), irradiation.

Clinical manifestations: white or discolored circumscribed flat patch may present fissuring, ulceration and induration.

Treatment: (a) elimination of a recognized causative factor; (b) multiple stage stripping; (c) topical application of vitamin A; (d) systemic management (hormone, vitamin).

C. LICHEN PLANUS

Etiology: unidentified (Grinspan's syndrome; lichen planus, diabetes mellitus, high arterial blood pressure).

Clinical manifestations: the various forms (plaque, vesicle, bulla, erosive, atrophic, hypertrophic) are all presenting the Wickham's striae radiating on their periphery and the small white dot at the intersection of these lines. Pruritus is characteristic.

Treatment: (a) watchful waiting to detect malignant transformation (repeated biopsy of a suspected area); (b) topical corticosteroids, tetracycline mouthwash, vitamin A, anesthetics; (c) systemic medications (vitamins, antidepressants, tranquilizers).

D. WHITE SPONGE NEVUS

Etiology: hereditary.

Clinical manifestations: asymptomatic, circumscribed, coarse opalescent corrugation, spongy texture.

Treatment: watchful waiting.

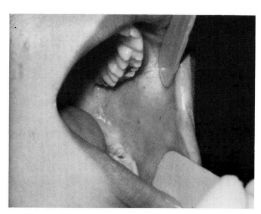

Figure 2.63 Inspection of the buccal region.

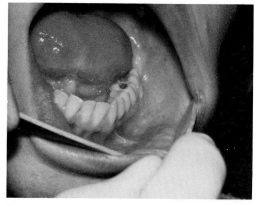

Figure 2.64 Inspection of the buccal vestibular area.

E. HEREDITARY BENIGN INTRAEPITHELIAL DYSKERATOSIS

Clinical manifestations: opalescent, spongy, coarse and macerated mucosa with sharp margins. Stretching the area presents elevated small plaques.
Treatment: watchful waiting.

F. LUPUS ERYTHEMATOSUS

Etiology: unknown.
Clinical manifestations: erythematous, asymptomatic, atrophic plaques, often with petechiae, hemorrhages, superficial painful ulcerations or crustings surrounded by keratotic margins, and hyperemic telangiectatic red halo.
Treatment: (a) corticosteroids; (b) antimalarial drugs.

G. ERYTHROPLAKIA

Etiology: unidentified.
Clinical manifestations: bright red plaque with well circumscribed margins, sometimes plaque of leukoplakia is present on the red base or small white spots ("speckled leukoplakia" or "speckled erythroplakia") are seen.
Treatment: (a) surgery; (b) irradiation.

H. INTRAEPITHELIAL AND INVASIVE EPIDERMOID CARCINOMA

Etiology: unidentified.
Clinical manifestations: plaque of leukoplakia, velvety erythroplakia, or leukoplakia on erythematous base. The development of thickened, raised, rolled margins, deep crater-like defect, irregular surface, granular, verrucous, exophytic or fungating proliferative neoplasm with fixation and induration; the almost invariable presence of ulceration (early, nontender, but ultimately painful) and regional lymph node metastasis.
Treatment: (a) surgery; (b) irradiation.

I. PAPILLOMA

Etiology: unknown.
Clinical manifestations: sessile or pedunculated verrucous benign tumor.
Treatment: surgical excision

J. FIBROMA

Etiology: unidentified.
Clinical manifestations: sessile or pedunculated, elevated, benign neoplasm with smooth surface, resilient to palpation.
Treatment: surgical excision.

K. MALIGNANT MELANOMA

Etiology: unknown.
Clinical manifestations: enlarging pigmented macules with outer erythematous zone, surface ulceration, haemorrhage and crustings.
Treatment: (a) surgical excision; (b) block dissection of regional lymph nodes.

L. LIPOMA

Etiology: unidentified.
Clinical manifestations: sessile or pedunculated, yellowish smooth surfaced, soft benign tumor.
Treatment: surgical excision.

M. OTHER ORAL LESIONS

Lesions presenting as specific and non-specific infections include Koplik's spots in measles, plaques of candidosis, noma, inflammatory (fibrous) hyperplasia, periadenitis mucosa necrotica recurrens, mucous retention phenomenon, recurrent aphthous ulcers, aspirin burns, stomatitis venenata, hematoma, ecchymosis, iatrogenic injuries, maceration of "pathomimia mucosae oris" are frequently encountered on this area.

Hard and Soft Palate

Tilt the head backwards to allow direct inspection of the roof of the mouth (Figures 2.66 and 2.67) by utilizing adequate light. Observe the appearance of rugae,

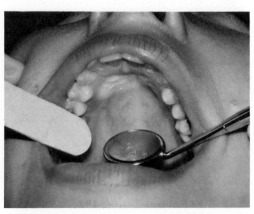

Figure 2.66 Inspection of the palate.

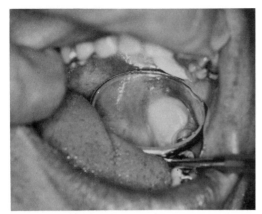

Figure 2.67 Inspection of the maxillary tuberosity region.

incisive papilla, palatal mucosa, vibration line, mobility of the soft palate and uvula (deviation), presence of postnasal discharge, developmental abnormalities (cleft palate, torus palatinus) fibrous masses and bony exostoses, asymmetries (sinus tumor), color changes. *Commonly seen abnormalities of the palate may include the following.*

A. INFLAMMATORY PAPILLARY HYPERPLASIA

Etiology: poor oral hygiene and denture irritation.

Clinical manifestations: numerous erythematous, edematous or normal colored fibromatous papillary projections of small sizes and various extent.

Treatment: (a) surgery; (b) elaboration of well-fitting denture(s).

B. TRAUMATIC ULCER

A bony spiculum may be left under the denture base, or the mucosal surface of the new denture has a "high" spot to initiate a decubital ulcer following the insertion of the denture. The treatment is "ironing-out" the bony spiculum, or remove the "high" spot of the denture.

C. STOMATITIS NICOTINA

Often observed in heavy pipe, cigar smokers, presenting multiple small nodules, each is covered by focal leukoplakia with a tiny erythematous dot on their center representing the inflamed minor palatal salivary duct opening.

Abnormalities of the Palate May Indicate:

1. Palatal spread of dental infection like palatal abscess following the periapical infection of a maxillary tooth and the development of an apical periodontal cyst.

2. Specific and nonspecific infection, such as syphilis, recurrent intraoral herpes simplex, herpangina, acute lymphonodular pharyngitis, hand, foot and mouth disease, herpes zoster, candidosis (denture sore mouth), pyogenic granuloma.

3. Developmental fissural cyst (median anterior maxillary cyst, median palatal cyst, globulomaxillary cyst).

4. Other disorders, including radiation mucositis of the palate, pizza burn and factitial injuries, denture base intolerance or allergic reactions, erythema multiforme group of lesions, pemphigoid, pemphigus, lichen planus, leukoplakia, benign and malignant neoplasms, erythroplakia, scarring.

Tongue

When the tongue is in a resting position, note the color (pink, pale, red, blue or yellow), the size, and the pattern of papillary distribution (filiform and fungiform papillae) on the dorsal surface of the tongue. When the patient places the tip of the tongue on the roof of the mouth, observe the mucosa of the ventral surface, the sublingual veins, the level of attachment of the lingual frenum (ankyloglossia) and the plicae fimbriatae (Figures 2.68 to 2.70). Follow the protrusive and lateral motions of the tongue, inspect the apex linguae. Note any deviation from expected

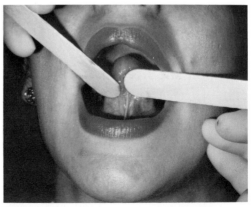

Figure 2.68 Inspecting the ventral surface of the tongue.

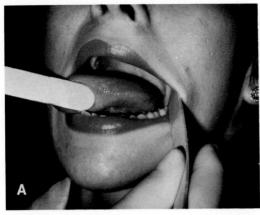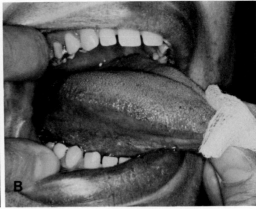

Figure 2.69   *A.* Inspecting the lateral surface of the tongue. *B.* Inspection of the foliate papillae region.

normal movements. Using 2 × 2 inch sterile gauze, extend the tongue anteriorly and laterally to see the appearance of the lateral margins and the most posterior parts of the tongue (the foliate and circumvallate papillae, some of the lingual tonsil of radix linguae). Palpate for tenderness, masses, texture and consistency, degree of hydration (moisture) and edema. Extend fissural patterns, crenations for close visualization. Scrape the dorsal surface with a tongue blade to see the amount of tongue coating. Describe the presence of abnormalities and lesions or the absence of filiform or fungiform papillae.

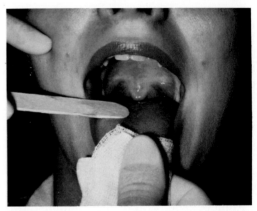

Figure 2.70   Inspecting the posterior part of the tongue.

Disorders Most Likely Seen on the Tongue

A. FISSURED TONGUE

Etiology: unidentified.

Clinical manifestations: various degree and extent of fissures, generally asymptomatic.

Treatment is restricted to cleansing of the fissures of the tongue and routine oral hygiene.

B. BENIGN MIGRATORY GLOSSITIS

Etiology: unidentified.

Clinical manifestations: circumscribed areas of desquamation of filiform papillae, persistence of fungiforms, surrounded by whitish margins and thin erythema. The denuded area may be sensitive spontaneously or by stimulation.

Treatment: symptomatic.

C. HAIRY TONGUE

Etiology: unidentified.

Clinical manifestations: excessive elongation of the filiform papillae usually covering the middle portion of the dorsal surface. The tongue coat is prominent around the hypertrophic papillae, the color of the region varies depending on exogenous discoloration.

Treatment: empirical, routine cleaning of the tongue. Application of podophyllin resin may be positive.

D. OROLINGUAL PARESTHESIA

Orolingual paresthesia (glossodynia, glossopyrosis), papilloma, fibroma, leukoplakia or erythoplakia, epidermoid carcinoma, localized phlebectasiae, hemangioma, lymphangioma, infections, nutritional deficiency, traumatic lesions, allergic reactions, erythema multiforme group of lesions, recurrent aphthous ulcers, lichen planus, etc., may be encountered during close lingual examination.

Floor of the Mouth

Have the patient elevate the tongue towards the roof of the mouth. Inspect the appearance of the soft tissues (shape, development, discoloration, hue, abnormalities) in the order of sublingual caruncles (the orifices of Wharton's ducts), sublingual folds (the Rivinus duct openings on the crest of the plicae), lingual alveolar mucosae, and the most posterior parts ("paralingual sulci") of the area (Figure 2.71). Palpate the entire floor of the mouth by using the bimanual technique for texture, moisture, unseen lumps, swelling masses and abnormal sores (Figure 2.72).

Some of the abnormalities of the floor of mouth are: leukoplakia; erythroplakia; various forms of lichen planus; ranula (retention cyst in association with Wharton's, Bartholin's or Rivinus ducts); mucocele (mucus retention phenomenon involving the minor salivary gland); submandibular sialolithiasis; symmetric swelling of dermoid or epidermoid cyst; oral lymphoepithelial cyst; purpuric manifestations of hematologic disorders; the white elevated soft plaques of candidosis; proliferative granulomatous, vegetative infection, widespread single or multiple ulcers of blasto-

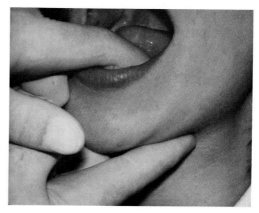

Figure 2.72 Bimanual palpation of the floor of the mouth.

mycosis (North and South American), coccidioidomycosis, histoplasmosis; recurrent aphthous ulcers; fiery red or catarrhal inflammation, small erosions, ulcers of scarlatina; irregular painful ulcers of various depths in tuberculosis; mucous patches, ulcers in syphilis; and epidermoid carcinoma and other neoplasms.

Pharynx

Observe the isthmus of the fauces, palatoglossal and palatopharyngeal arches, tonsillar fossae, palatal tonsils present, enlargements, asymmetries, color of mucous membranes, inflammation, exudate and character, granulation tissue, ulceration, and other lesions.

A. OROPHARYNX (MESOPHARYNX)

Depressing the tongue base by tongue blade while the patient says "Ah" permits the sight of any disorder (color, masses, lesions, purpura) of the lateral and posterior walls of the pharynx, the (Figure 2.73) motion of palate and uvula. Note the presence of "gag reflex," be prepared to quickly relieve the patient from this phase of the examination in case of "hyperreflexia."

B. NASOPHARYNX (EPIPHARYNX)

Extend the patient's tongue gently by using gauze. Introduce a slightly warmed hand (dental) mirror without touching the soft tissues of the isthmus (avoid gag reflex). Project light into the nasopharyngeal

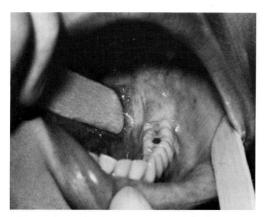

Figure 2.71 Inspection of the most posterior portion of the floor of the mouth.

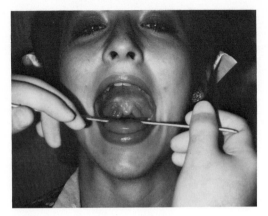

Figure 2.73 Inspection of the oropharynx (while the patient says "Ah").

area. Inspect the posterior choanae, nasal septum, discharge, pharyngeal tonsils (adenoids), Rosenmüller fossae.

C. LARYNGOPHARYNX (HYPOPHARYNX)

Protrude the tongue by the gauze technique. Introduce the mirror as described above and project the light into the laryngopharynx ("indirect laryngoscopy") (Figure 2.74). Observe the lingual tonsil area and the entire base of the tongue, the patency of piriform recesses, the epiglottis. Describe any symptom of difficult swallowing or "lump in the throat," spots of tenderness, sores, "full feeling," or "tightness" in the throat, the presence of nodules or masses, the places where solid food "sticks," regurgitation of liquids, general "sore throat" sensation, character of the voice (hoarseness, decrease in loudness, change in pitch, aphonia or loss of voice), cough with sputum production (frequency, amount and character).

Some of the following lesions may be seen during the examination of the pharyngeal area: tonsillitis, adenoiditis, pharyngitis due to *bacterial infections* ("strep" throat, stomatitis scarlatina, tuberculosis usually secondary to pulmonary involvement, diphtheritic membrane); *viral disease* (diffuse inflammation, small discrete vesicles, multiple ulcers in measles, rubella, primary herpetic stomatitis, varicella, herpes zoster, hand, foot and mouth disease, generalized sore throat in viral hepatitis; single, elevated whitish papules

surrounded by narrow erythematous zone in acute lymphonodular pharyngitis); *mycotic infections* (firm masses at the radix linguae in botryomycosis; white monilial plaque (thrush) of candidiasis; soft vascular, erythematous, purpuric growths with mucopurulent exudate in rhinosporidiosis; nonspecific ulcerations and soft scar formation in sporotrichosis), recurrent aphthous ulcers, periadenitis mucosa necrotica recurrens (large painful ulcers and scarring), lesions of erythema exudative multiforme, Stevens-Johnson syndrome, hemorrhages related to hematologic disorders, lingual thyroid nodule, glossopharyngeal neuralgia (periodic sharp pain), scleroderma (stiff throat sensation), neoplasms (squamous cell carcinoma of the naso-orolaryngopharynx, malignant reticuloendotheliosis/Wegner's granulomatosis, nasopharyngeal angiofibroma, malignant lymphoma, etc.), hoarseness (rule out neoplastic involvement of the recurrent laryngeal nerve).

Gingivae and Alveolar Mucosae

Inspect the gingivae at various locations; papillary, cervical, attached, incisive, retromolar, the mucogingival relationship and the alveolar mucosae, the frenal (labial, buccal, lingual) attachments, the general architecture (recession of the gingival margin), swelling (hypertrophy, hyperplasia), color and hue. *Palpate* the tone, texture, tenderness. Record abnormal pigmentation (may vary widely depending on the level of racial skin pigmentation), inflammatory lesions, desquama-

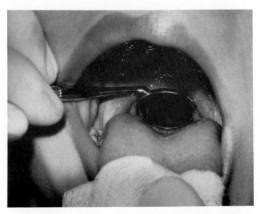

Figure 2.74 Indirect laryngoscopy.

tions, bleeding and necrosis. Measure the depth of pockets present.

Gingival and alveolar mucosal disorders may be discovered during examination, including the following: inflammatory and noninflammatory (fibrous) hyperplasia as in endocrine imbalance (puberty, pregnancy, hyperparathyroidism), regional enteritis (Crohn's disease), scurvy, Dilantin; fibromatosis gingivae; chronic desquamative gingivitis (benign mucous membrane pemphigoid); lupus erythematosus; lichen planus; leukoplakia; erythroplakia; papilloma; lipoma; fibroma; peripheral giant cell granuloma; squamous cell carcinoma, melanocarcinoma and other neoplasms; odontogenic cysts and tumors; nonspecific infections of the periapical tissues; specific infections (tuberculosis, acute necrotizing ulcerative gingivitis, herpes simplex); periodontal diseases; recurrent aphthous ulcers; pemphigus, hematologic disorders; pigmented cellular nervus; traumatic ulcer; allergy.

Jaw Bones and Alveoli

Observe the size and shape of the jaws, use the dental mirror to see the hidden sites, e.g., posterolateral part of the maxillary tuberosity and the most posterior aspect of the lingual surface of the mandible. Palpate for tenderness, swelling, fluctuation, crepitation and discharge. Evaluate the roentgenographic findings. Lesions that may be seen in association with these bones are the following: periodontal disease, diseases of the periapical tissues (periapical granuloma, apical periodontal cyst, periapical abscess, osteomyelitis), developmental/fissural cysts, gnathoschisis, palatoschisis, micrognathia, macrognathia, odontogenic cysts and tumors, other neoplasms (chondroma, osteoma, sarcoma, malignant lymphoma, multiple myeloma, solitary plasma cell myeloma, metastases of the jaws), tori and bony exostoses, central ossifying fibroma of bone, central giant cell granuloma, central hemangioma of bone, aneurysmal bone cyst, traumatic cyst, fractures, cherubism, fibrous dysplasia of bone, developmental lingual mandibular salivary gland depression, granulomatous inflammatory lesions due to specific infections, disostoses (cleidocranial, craniofacial, mandibulofacial), osteope-

trosis, osteitis deformans, hyperparathyroidism.

Teeth

Inspection of the number, location, degree of eruption and the dental age, shade, size, shape, contact points, functional (masticatory) relationship, occlusion, degree of tooth abrasion, level of oral hygiene condition (plaque, calculus, intensity of halitosis), and of the individual teeth: discoloration (extrinsic stain, e.g., tobacco; intrinsic stain, e.g., tetracycline—use the UV light), malposition (malocclusion), migration, diastemas, malformation and deformity, caries, degree of gingival recession, inflammation and the state of dental restorations and appliances. *Palpate* for decay, sensitivity (tooth neck), pockets, fremitus and tooth mobility. *Percuss* for sensitivity. Investigate for impaction, fracture, cavity, level of the alveolar bone by using roentgenographs. Look out for the following disorders: dental caries and its consequences, periodontal disease, attrition, abrasion, erosion, embedded and impacted teeth, odontogenic cysts and tumors, cementum hyperplasia, dilated composite odontoma, enamel hypoplasia, enamel hypomineralization, amelogenesis imperfecta, dentinal dysplasia, dentinogenesis imperfecta, gemination, fusion, concrescence, talon cusp, dilaceration, taurodontism, tooth ankylosis, external or internal root resorption, supernumerary roots and cusps, supernumerary teeth, microdontia, macrodontia, anodontia, delayed eruption, premature eruption (Figures 2.75 to 2.77).

Session Three: Emergency Dental Examination

An emergency is defined as an unforeseen combination of occurrences which require immediate attention to be rectified. An emergency evaluation as related to disorders of oral soft and hard tissue is limited. It is directly associated with signs and symptoms of the patient's chief complaint, the relevant disease process and its likely etiology. The ultimate success of the emergency case history and examination is di-

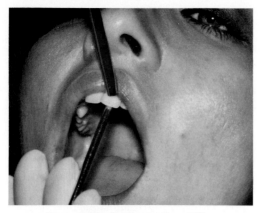

Figure 2.75   Testing tooth mobility.

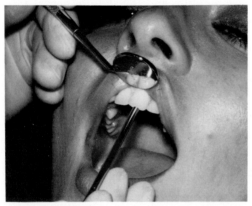

Figure 2.76   Percussion of the tooth (parallel).

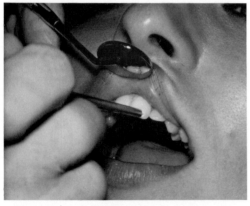

Figure 2.77   Percussion of the tooth (angular).

rectly related to the examiner's ability to utilize effectively the basic principles of oral medicine/diagnosis, namely, interviewing, performing adequate clinical examination and arriving at a diagnosis quickly. The emphasis is placed upon the

evaluation of acute and known complaints that may serve to provide the examiner with sufficient information to establish an "immediate" diagnosis and to institute the appropriate treatment, or relief of symptoms. In the emergency type of examination, existing circumstances determine the trend of the examination. The rationale of diagnosis is based on systematic observation and a logical description of manifestations of the disease. The following table (Table 2.2) consists of the simplest forms of emergency dental examination involving oral hard tissues. The facts gathered in the history and the presence or absence of signs and symptoms should orient the dentist's thinking to the basic mechanisms responsible for the existing disease. The method of clinical examination is supplemented by inspection of radiographs and other tests, in order to determine the causative disease in the patient.

Dental emergencies may include the following disorders.

Acute Periapical Abscess. The tooth is extremely painful, slightly extruded; regional lymphadenitis and fever may be present; slight thickening of the periodontal membrane may be seen on the roentgenograph. Treatment: antibiotic, drainage.

Acute Osteomyelitis. Loose, sore tooth; severe pain; regional lymphadenopathy; fever; leukocytosis; diffuse osteolytic changes may be seen on the roentgenograph in two weeks. Treatment: drainage, antibiotics.

Acute Periostitis. The findings are related to the osteomyelitis; reddening and swelling of the covering membranes is characteristic. Therapy: similar to that of the osteomyelitis.

Phlegmon (Cellulitis). Firm, diffuse, painful swelling of the inflamed soft tissues, fistulous tract may be seen, regional lymphadenopathy, leukocytosis, fever. Treatment: antibiotics.

Ludwig's Angina. Painful, rapidly developing diffuse, firm swelling of the floor of the mouth, elevation of the tongue, involvement of the submandibular space, difficult respiration, fever, rapid pulse and respiratory rate, leukocytosis. Treatment: antibiotics, sometimes coniotomy or tracheotomy.

Acute Pericoronitis. Fluctuant abscess

Table 2.2
Emergency Dental Examination

Diagnosis	Inspection	Sensitivity to			Radiograph	EPT[a]	Sensitivity to		Pain	Osmosis (sweet, sour)	Transillu-mination	Treatment
		Percus-sion	Palpation	Mobility			Cold	Heat				
Hyperemia of pulp	Caries	–	–	–	+	d	+	–	Short, sharp, parox-ysmal	+	–	Sedative dress-ing
Acute serous pulpitis	Caries	–	–	–	+	d	+	–	Sharp, throbbing, paroxysmal or continuous	+	–	Pulp extirpation
Acute suppura-tive pulpitis	Caries	+ (In later stage)	–	–	+	d: early i: late	+	+	Intermittent (early), dull (late), throbbing (late), constant	–	–	Pulp extirpation
Acute apical periodontitis	Caries	+	+	+	+ (Occlusal trauma) (vi-tal)	n or –	–	–	–	–	+	Disocclusion, drainage
Acute alveolar abscess	May have ele-vated tempera-ture, fistula	+ (Se-vere)	+ (Swell-ing)	+	+ –	slight or –	– +	+ –		–	+	Disocclusion, drainage, anti-biotic

[a] d = decreased threshold
i = increased threshold
n = normal threshold

formation, inflammatory edema, pain, regional lymphadenopathy, fever, malaise. Therapy: drainage, antibiotics.

Acute Periodontal Abscess. Sudden subperiosteal pus accumulation over the root surface, at the gingival area; tender, mobile, tooth. Treatment: drainage.

Allergic Reactions. May consist of the most frequent emergency complications encountered in the dental office.

Acute Maxillary Sinusitis. Continuous, throbbing ache at infraorbital region may be related to postural change, multiple maxillary odontalgia, fever, nasal or postnasal discharge, cloudiness on radiograph. Therapy: antibiotics, analgesics, vasoconstrictors, drainage.

Temporomandibular Joint Pain. Diffuse pain in preauricular area accompanied by acute pain during mandibular movements. Therapy: analgesics, tranquilizers, relative immobilization of the mandible.

Session Four: Radiographs

The usual routine is to make the following radiographs during the examination of the dental patients: periapical, bite-wing and panoramic (if available).

The indication for radiographs at the time of reexamination depends on several factors judged by the clinician, including the level of oral hygiene of the patient, e.g., poor oral hygiene may necessitate periodic checks every few months, while good oral hygiene may allow a few years between radiographic examinations. The existing diagnostic and therapeutic factors should be considered in deciding the proper time intervals between radiographic examinations, e.g., evaluation of a periapical area every six months subsequent to the completion of endodontic therapy, or the "watchful waiting" in the presence of, e.g., monostotic fibrous dysplasia of the jaw.

1. The intraoral *periapical* radiographs (Figure 2.78)—either the paralleling technique or the bisecting-angle technique— are used to view the teeth, including the roots, the periapical regions and the structures of the surrounding alveolar areas.

The central ray should be aimed to pass through the region to be examined and the film packet should be positioned so that it will record that region with minimal distortion in the central portion of the film.

2. *Bite-wing* (Figure 2.79) radiographs should provide good views of proximal surfaces of the posterior teeth, e.g., proximal caries, the anatomy of the pulp chamber, the pulpal horns and orifices of root canals, the crests of both interdental and interradicular alveolar septi, e.g., periodontal disease. This technique is less frequently utilized for the examinations of anterior teeth.

3. *Panoramic* (Figure 2.80) radiography permits the survey of the entire maxilla and mandible, including the temporomandibular joints, the maxillary sinuses, nasal cavity and turbinate bones, the nasal septum, hard palate, the mandibular condyles, rami and dentoalveolar regions. The panoramic view of the dentition is advantageous in rapid assessment of dental status and treatment planning.

The following radiographic techniques have rather specialized indications:

4. The *occlusal* (Figure 2.81) radiographs of the mandible or the maxilla are invaluable in examining the mediolateral extension of structures located in the

   a. Mandible: floor of the mouth (e.g., to reveal a sialolith in Wharton's duct). (1) Anterior portion of the mandible (e.g., fracture or localizing foreign bodies). (2) Posterior portion of the mandible (e.g., retained roots, osteoslcerosis).

   b. Maxilla: the hard palate and the anterior regions of the maxilla (e.g., cysts, unerupted teeth). Provides a good view of the floor of the maxillary sinus.

5. Extraoral *lateral jaw* (Figure 2.82) roentgenographs are indicated to view the body of the mandible, to examine premolar and molar areas and the mandibular ramus, to identify sialoliths in the submandibular/sublingual salivary glands or ducts and to localize foreign bodies and displaced roots near the mandible. Standard lateral views are helpful, when indicated, in studying the right or left temporomandibular joints, either with the patient's teeth in occlusion or with the mouth wide open.

6. The *Waters* view (Figure 2.83) (posteroanterior oblique projection) is indicated to demonstrate the maxillary and

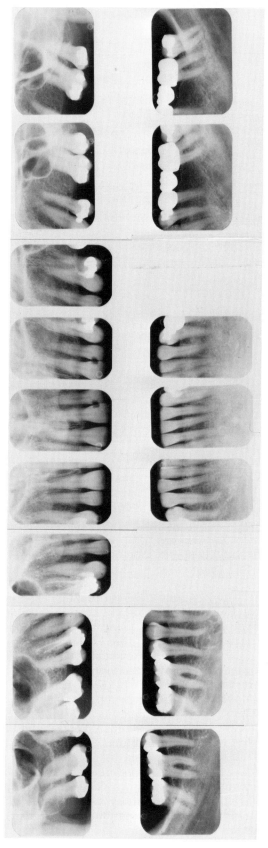

Figure 2.78 Periapical radiographs.

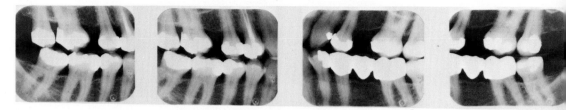

Figure 2.79 Bite-wing radiographs.

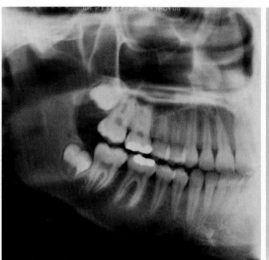
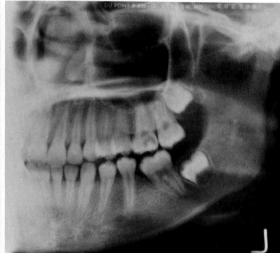

Figure 2.80 Panoramic radiographs.

frontal sinuses, maxillary frontal processes, supraorbital and infraorbital ridges, nasal bones, cellulae mastoideae, zygomatic bones and arches, condylar and coronoid processes and the mandibular angles.

7. *Towne's* projection (Figure 2.84) (anteroposterior view) shows the condylar and styloid processes, temporomandibular joints (the teeth are in occlusion), angles of the mandible, the rami of the mandible, the medial aspects of the pterygopalatine fossae, nasal septum and turbinate bones, sphenoidal sinus (superimposed on the foramen occipitale magnum).

8. *Submental-vertex* (Figure 2.85) to project the zygomatic arches is indicated to demonstrate fractures, foreign bodies and basilar skull structures.

9. *Oblique lateral transcranial projection* (Figure 2.86) is oriented to view the structures of the temporomandibular joint of one side.

10. *Lateral projection of nasal bones* (Figure 2.87) shows the nasal bones, maxillary frontal processes and anterior nasal spine.

11. The *lateral* (Figure 2.88) and *posteroanterior skull* (Figure 2.89) projections are useful to study the radiographic anatomy of the head in both mediolateral and anteroposterior directions, respectively; these radiographs may also represent cephalometric radiographic views for orthodontic purposes.

12. *Sialography* (Figure 2.90) is indicated to view salivary gland structures, the duct patterns, the function of the salivary glands involved, and their pathologic conditions. It is customary to support the finding by a further diagnostic radiographic method: *sequential salivary scintigraphy*.

13. *Cinefluorography* is indicated to study movements of the temporomandibular joints and the structures of mastication and deglutition.

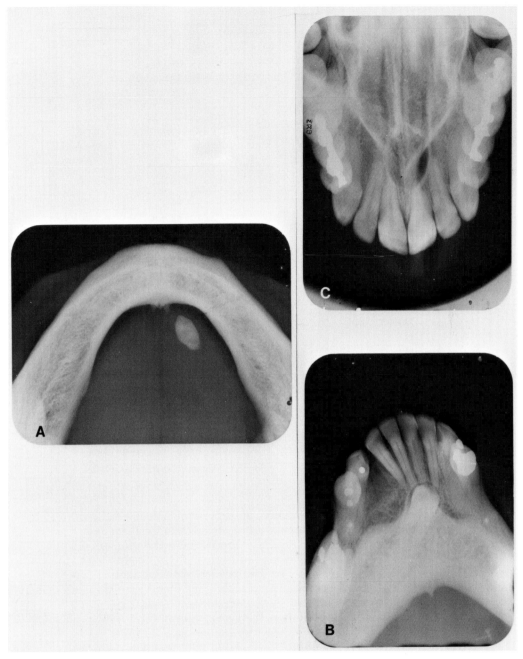

Figure 2.81 Occlusal radiographs. *A*. Mandible—floor of the mouth (sialolith in Wharton's duct). *B*. Anterior portion of the mandible (impacted canine). *C*. Maxilla (cyst development).

Session Five: Diagnostic Tests

Diagnosis or confirmation of a diagnosis many times depends on proper laboratory tests.

Laboratory procedures and services may be grouped into: blood chemistry, hema- tology, immunology, urinalysis, histopa- thology and cytology, bacteriology, etc., serving as useful diagnostic mechanisms for evaluating pathoses. The dentist should be familiar with many of these testing procedures, have a reasonable justification for ordering tests, be able to interpret their result and intelligently communicate with

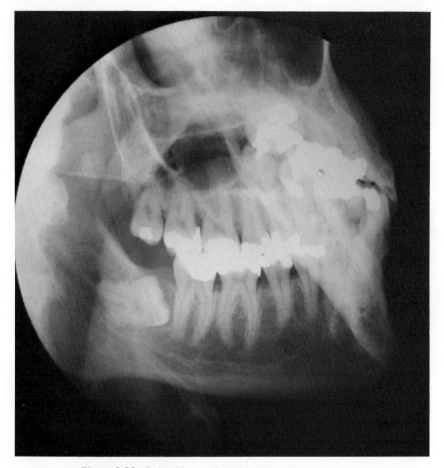

Figure 2.82 Lateral jaw radiographs (impacted third molar).

all others involved in the patient's care, and determine the influence of systemic factors on oral diseases so that patient management will be based on a knowledge of the etiology of disease rather than on therapy aimed only by treating symptoms.

Some of the more common laboratory screening procedures or tests to diagnose specific abnormalities will be discussed in this section. Using automated techniques, multiple hematology and blood chemistry tests are now available at very low cost and are performed with reasonable accuracy.

Normal values are considered those that fall within two standard deviations from the mean (about 95% of the population).

Normal values vary with the method employed, the laboratory, the conditions of specimen collection and preservation;

always consult the given laboratory to obtain their normal values.

Proper interpretation of laboratory results must always be related to the clinical condition of the patient.

Capillary blood may be used for hemoglobin or hemotocrit cell counts, blood typing, coagulation time or microchemical determinations.

Following is a list of laboratory procedures included.

1. Microhematocrit
2. Bleeding time
3. Capillary fragility
4. Venipuncture
5. Clot retraction
6. Blood clotting
7. Erythrocyte sedimentation rate
8a. Sequential multiple analysis 12
8b. Sequential multiple analysis 16

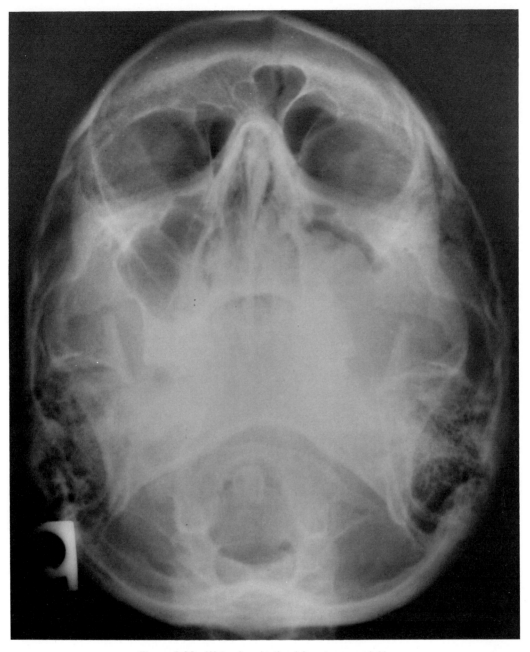

Figure 2.83 Waters' projection (sinus tumor on left).

9. Blood glucose
10. Urinalysis
11. Occult blood in stool
12. Smear for light microscopic examination
13. Microbiologic culture and/or animal inoculation
14. Biopsy
15. Normal hematologic values

1. Microhematocrit

This test is used for the detection of anemia. Anemia is a symptom, a sign of an underlying disease, it is not a disease or diagnosis per se. Anemia is defined as a decrease in the amount of oxygen carrying hemoglobin (Hb) per unit volume of blood (normal range of Hb concentration is: male

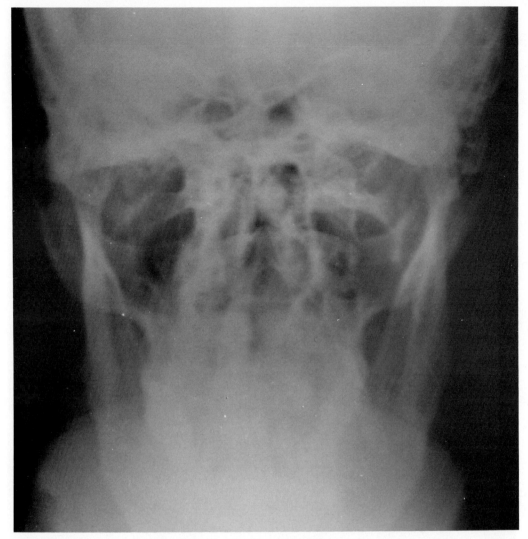

Figure 2.84   Towne's projection.

12 to 17 gm%, female 11 to 15 gm%) which may be the result of a pathologic decrease in the red cell count (normal RBC: male 4.5 to 6.0 $\times$ 10^6/mm^3; female 4.0 to 5.5 $\times$ 10^6/mm^3). Since the mature RBCs are fully saturated with hemoglobin such a decrease means a reduction in total blood hemoglobin concentration.

Anemia may be detected by RBC count, blood smear, Hb concentration or hematocrit (Hct).

Hct can be detected from a finger prick. This is known as microhematocrit. The microhematocrit is well adapted for dental office use.

Indications: Signs and symptoms of anemia include pallor, dyspnea, tachycardia, Hx of excessive or frequent blood loss, pale oral mucous membrane, conjunctiva, nail beds, skin, unexplained syncope (not vasovagal or hypoglycemic), excessive fatigue, atrophy of lingual papillae, glossitis, gingival hemorrhages, stomatitis, excessive bruising and petechial hemorrhages. *Routine:* prior to general anesthesia and surgery. It is important to know if the reduction of transported oxygen is expected, or if hemorrhage is expected during surgery which could aggravate the anemia present.

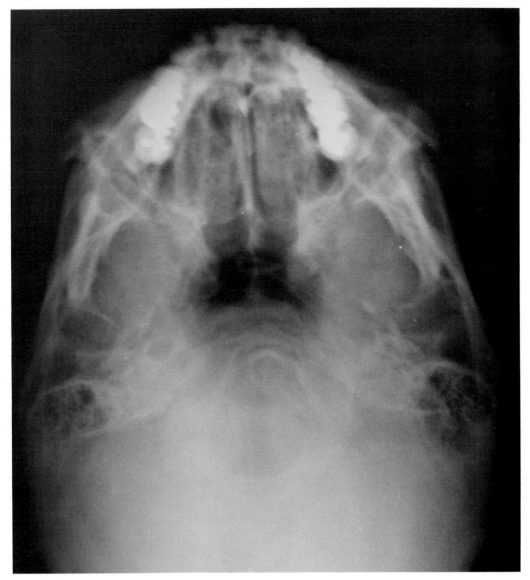

Figure 2.85 Submental-vertex projection.

Procedure:

a. Hold finger (big toe of babies) without compressing it, clean with 70% alcohol sponges and allow to dry.

b. Prick the dry finger with the lancet (the entire point of a 2 mm lancet to the stop is used to assure adequate blood flow).

c. Wipe away the first drop and fill two heparinized capillary tubes with blood that wells up freely (mix the anticoagulant with blood slowly to avoid hemolysis).

d. Don't compress finger to avoid dilution with connective tissue fluid and hold the capillary downward.

e. Seal one end with clay (Critoseal).

f. Centrifuge for five minutes at 12,000 rpm.

g. Read hematocrit by sliding capillary tube so that the outer end of the tube is on "0" and the air-serum interface is on "100." This is achieved by turning the head plate. Volume of packed red blood cells (Hct) expressed as a percentage of

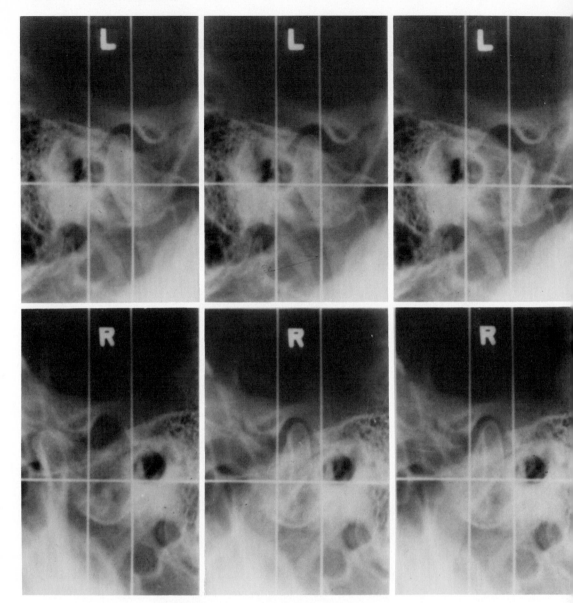

Figure 2.86   Oblique lateral transcranial projections (TMJ).

a sample of whole blood (the whole blood volume is essentially composed of RBC and plasma).

Interpretation: microhematocrit (an index of the erythrocyte count) is as accurate as macrohematocrit, normal Hct: male 40 to 54%, female 37 to 47%. (The average error is about 1 to 2%.) Reduced: mild—hemodilution; severe—anemia (necessary to do a complete blood count). Increased: mild—hemoconcentration; severe—polycythemia, tuberculosis, neoplasm.

Buffy coat: a 0.5 mm-thick, whitish layer over the RBC column; it contains WBC and platelets. Its thickness increases in leukocytosis (platelet never increases that much to increase its thickness significantly). Less than 0.5 mm packed white blood cells indicates a leukopenia. Increased: infection, neoplasm. In case of leukemia the buffy coat may be several millimeters thick.

The supernatant (plasma) of the Hct tube is of straw color; if yellow: increased bilirubin (icterus index); if red: hemolysis; if milky: elevated plasma lipids.

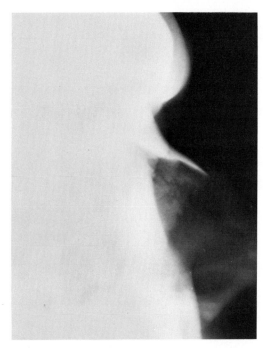

Figure 2.87 Lateral projection of nasal bones.

2. Bleeding Time

The history of a patient may reveal prolonged bleeding following extraction, and spontaneous bleeding, petechial hemorrhages, easy bruising or multiple transfusions after surgery. *Bleeding time* (Ivy technique) is a good screening test to provide information for further detailed hematologic workup. It is a measure of blood vessel retractability and defects in platelets, either in number or in functional ability.

Indications: Hx of previous bleeding, abnormal microhematocrit, primary screening test for disorders of hemostasis. Bleeding time may be prolonged in disorders of hemostatic mechanisms, but patient may have severe bleeding with normal time (e.g., hemophiliacs have no problems with small cuts because of the extrinsic mechanism).

Procedure:

a. Place sphygmomanometer cuff above elbow and inflate to 40 mm Hg (to standardize technique).
b. Clean volar surface with alcohol and allow to dry.
c. Tense skin of forearm by grasping the arm between the thumb and forefinger (select an area free of superficial veins).

d. Pierce skin to a depth of 4 mm with blood lancet (Sera-Sharp).
e. Absorb for 30 seconds on edge of filter paper.
f. At end of 1 minute make another puncture 1 cm from the first (to check on the other).
g. Continue to absorb the blood on the filter paper at 30-sec intervals until bleeding ceases (ignore oozing of blood tinged fluid).

If arm shows cyanosis, release pressure intermittently. Discontinue test if petechiae, ecchymoses appear.

Interpretation: normal values 6 to 10 minutes; should the bleeding continue beyond 15 minutes discontinue test. In many patients the first drop may be small due to vasoconstriction. Increased: idiopathic thrombocytopenia (Werlhof)—secondary purpura (2° to marrow destruction, drug sensitivity, chronic hepatitis, late renal disease, thrombotic thrombocytopenia); pseudohemophilia (Willebrand)—e.g., 300 minutes; vascular disorders (defective capillary wall function); thrombasthenia (Glanzmann's disease); severe defect in thromboplastin generation; may be positive in severe defect of thrombogenesis (heparin therapy) or fibrin formation.

3. Capillary Fragility (Tourniquet, Rumpel-Leede) Test

Indications: spontaneous bruising; thrombocytopenia (moderate 100,000/mm^3; severe 50,000/mm^3) idiopathic thrombocytopenic purpura (ITP), secondary (immunologic or drug-induced) thrombocytopenia; intrinsic defect in capillary wall (vascular purpura)—scurvy, collagen diseases, petechiae in the oral cavity and skin.

Procedure:

a. Petechiae preexisting on the skin are marked with ink.
b. Sphygmomanometer cuff is inflated above the elbow, midway between systolic and diastolic pressure, 120/60 = 90, but should not exceed 100 mm Hg, e.g., 160/90 for 10 minutes.
c. Use diascopy to test the developed spot (in telangiectasia the blood is intravascular and blanching).
d. Note development of petechiae in a 2.5

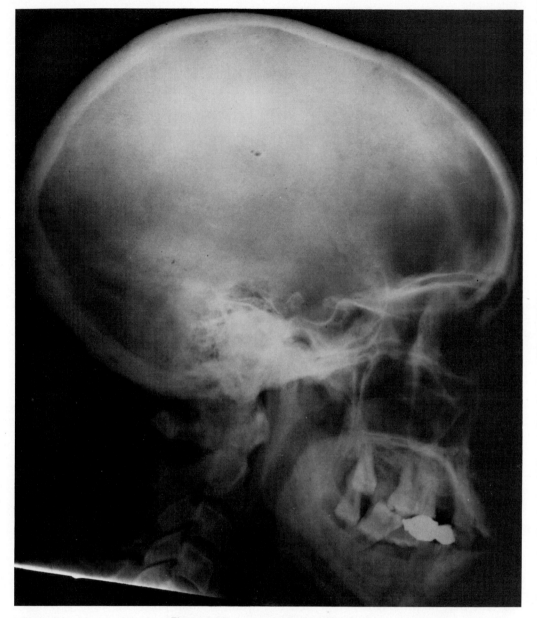

Figure 2.88 Lateral skull projection.

cm circle: negative 0 (no extravasation, no petechiae).

+1

++10

+++20

++++50

Remember: before proceeding with this test examine the oral cavity and skin for petechiae, and if petechiae are present nothing will be gained by performing this test and severe petechial disfiguring may occur.

Interpretation: testing the ability of superficial skin capillaries to withstand an increased intraluminal pressure, a degree of hypoxia or anoxia developing by the short term occlusion of veins. The blood vessels of normal patient withstand this condition and no petechiae develop.

False positive result: patient is conva-

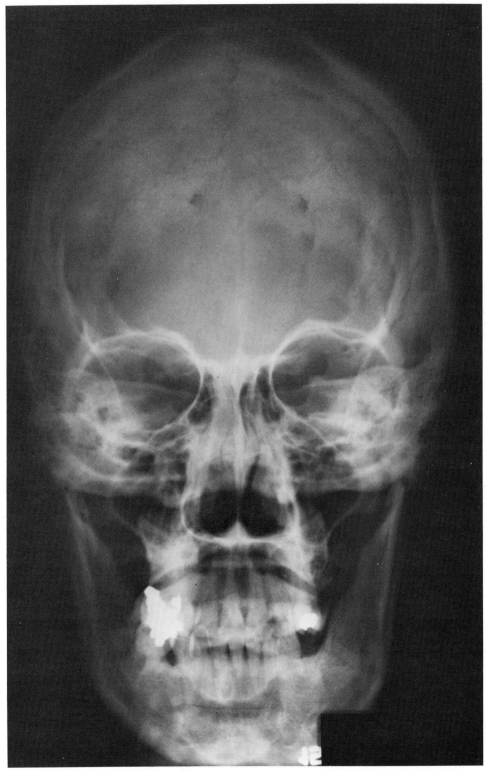

Figure 2.89 Posteroanterior skull projection.

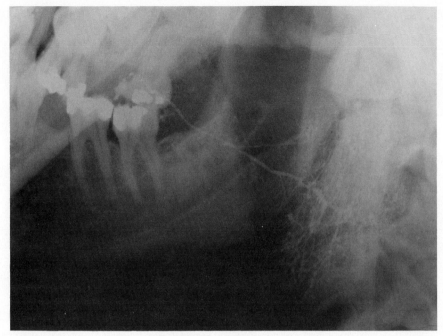

Figure 2.90 Sialography.

lescing from an infection (URI); allergies; elderly, red-haired women.

The test is positive: idiopathic thrombocytopenia (Werlhof); fibrinogenopenia; pseudohemophilia; 2° purpura (vascular types of purpura, drug sensitivity, bone marrow destructions, chronic liver disease, late renal disease, hereditary and thrombotic thrombocytopenia); arthritis, collagen disease; bleeding, bruising Hx; septicemia; erythematous infections; Henoch-Schönlein purpura; senile purpura, scurvy.

Negative for hemophilia (factor VIII, IX, XI deficiency).

4. Venipuncture

Many hematological tests, e.g., CBC, serology and clinical chemical determinations, are performed on samples of venous rather than capillary blood. Venous blood is usually obtained from an antecubital vein. Sterile needle and syringe are necessary. The best way for sterilization is by means of an autoclave (7.8 kg, 121°C, 15 minutes, need to put stylets into wrap parts). Note: dry them, since wetness will cause hemolysis; or use dry heat (180° C, 30 minutes). Use 20 or 21 gauge needles

(siliconized) for routine collection. Sterile disposable needles and syringes are preferred. Sealed evacuated containers (*Vacutainer tubes*) are available (Table 2.3).

Multiple sample needles are used for multiple specimens (plastic sleeve on the short part of the double pointed needle). The needle is held by a plastic cylindrical cap.

Procedure:
a. Apply tourniquet and select vein, ask patient to close and open fist repeatedly.
b. Apply alcohol (70%), air dry.
c. Fix the skin with one hand and insert needle into vein: keep 30° angle with skin; if the vein is small orient the needle as shown.

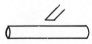

if the vein is large insert the needle like this.

d. Aspirate blood.

Table 2.3
Use of Venipuncture

Indications	Stopper Color	Volume of Tube	Tube Contents
Serologies (antibodies, e.g., rubella test, VDRL) Enzymes chemistries (SMA$_{12}$, SMA$_6$) (Use slide smear for differential blood count); T$_3$T$_4$	Red	10, 15 ml	Empty
Hematology Hb Platelet adhesiveness Hb electrophoresis; chemistries (not for electrolytes and nonprotein nitrogen)	Lavender	7 ml	EDTA
Prothrombin Partial thromboplastin	Black	4.5 ml	Sodium citrate
Blood glucose Fibrinogen	Blue	4.5 ml	Fluoride and oxalate (fluoride inhibits glycolysis for hours)
Corticosteroids sp. hematology	Green	10 ml	Na heparin
SGOT Blood glucose GTT BUN Prothrombin	Gray	10 ml	Oxalate
ANA LE prep Rh typing Blood typing	Yellow	4.5 ml	Silicone smoky side

e. Release tourniquet.

f. Place dry cotton over puncture and withdraw needle, bring patient's arm in flexion and let patient elevate the arm to prevent extravasation of blood.

If syncope/hematoma develops, loosen tourniquet and remove needle; try the other arm.

All the specimens should be delivered to the laboratory in a few hours or may be kept at 4°C (do not freeze this blood specimen) overnight.

Consult the laboratory for the *required Vacutainer tube*, always ask for their normal values.

Note: treat the blood gently to minimize hemolysis when mixing in the tube.

5. Clot Retraction

No anticoagulant; failure of blood to retract may indicate thrombocytopenia, idiopathic thrombocytopenia; secondary purpura; fibrinogen deficit; thrombasthenia.

6. Blood Clotting (Coagulation)

Plasma: has components of coagulation proteins. Serum: obtained after coagulation (clotting), clear, straw colored. Failure of blood to coagulate within 20 minutes may indicate hemophilia or other coagulation (prothrombin complex deficit, fibrinogen deficiency, heparin therapy) defects, and the need for further tests. Normal: 10 to 18 minutes by using Wassermann tube.

Prothrombin time (PT) and partial thromboplastin time (PTT) are tests of the coagulation phase. Together these two tests would detect 95% of coagulation disorders.

CURRENT THEORY OF BLOOD COAGULATION STAGES

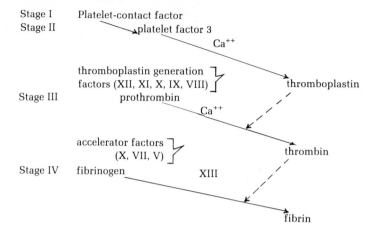

Prothrombin time (Quick's method, PT). Prothrombin is essential in blood clotting. It is abnormal in vitamin K deficiency, hepatitis and biliary diseases. The following is a brief description of the technic.

a. Take 4.5 ml venous blood and 0.5 ml sodium oxalate and centrifuge 15 min. at 3000 rpm.

b. Place plasma, thromboplastin solution and calcium chloride solution (1.11%) in water bath at 37°C (98.6°F).

c. Add 0.1 ml of plasma to 0.1 ml of thromboplastin solution in a hemolysis tube; quickly add 0.1 ml of calcium chloride solution and start stopwatch.

d. Note the time in seconds as soon as plasma no longer flows. Normal prothrombin time: 16 seconds; 60 to 100%.

The PT is not influenced by stage I and II defects since a complete thromboplastin reagent is provided.

Increased: anticoagulant therapy (heparin, coumarins); fibrinogen deficit; prothrombin complex deficiency; factor VII deficiency.

Decreased: pseudohemophilia (Willebrand).

Partial thromboplastin time (PTT). A partial ("incomplete"—essentially a platelet substitute lacking all other thromboplastin components) thromboplastin reagent plus calcium is added to the plasma in the same way as the PT.

Interpretation: highly positive in stage II defects; stage I abnormality doesn't influence the PTT; may be abnormal in severe stage III and IV defects.

Coagulation Disorders: deficiency of factors VIII, IX, XI, or XII; deficiency of factor VII; deficiencies of factors V, X, prothrombin or fibrinogen. Hereditary coagulation defects are usually single and persist throughout life; the concentration of a deficient factor may vary from a trace to 60%. In coagulation disorders, the coagulation time is abnormal while the bleeding time is usually normal.

7. Erythrocyte Sedimentation Rate (ESR)

Normal ESR does not exclude the possibility of disease, but an altered rate is an indication for further study. It is a nonspecific parameter of inflammation. (The rate in the female is increased because of steroids: male—10 mm/hr; female—20 mm/hr.

An altered albumin/globulin ratio: increased albumin, fibrinogen and decreased albumin will result in increased ESR.

The Westergren, Wintrobe methods: a 100-mm long, graduated hematocrit tube in a vertical position containing anticoagulant is used. Mixing should be complete, but care must be taken to prevent foaming.

Rapid (high ESR): menstruation; extensive inflammation, cell destruction, toxemia; rheumatoid arthritis; pregnancy, puerperium; active rheumatic fever; nephrosis; acute myocardial infarction; shock; syphilis; postoperative states; acute or chronic infections; tuberculosis; appendicitis, salpingitis; necrotic, infected malignant tumors; liver disease (cirrhosis).

Slow (low ESR): allergic conditions; polycythemia; congestive heart failure; sickle cell anemia; newborn.

8. SMA₁₂ and SMA₆

Table 2.4 provides a serum analysis of the SMA₁₂ and SMA₆ tests.

INTERPRETATION OF SEQUENTIAL MULTIPLE ANALYZER-12 TEST (STANDARD SMA₁₂)

Elevated Cholesterol. Cholesterol metabolism is intimately associated with lipid metabolism; chronic hepatitis, biliary cirrhosis, biliary obstruction, arteriosclerosis, cardiovascular disease, diabetes mellitus, obesity, nephrosis, pregnancy, lipemia, hypoproteinemia, familial hypercholesterolemia, hypothyroidism (myxedema, cretinism), hypopituitarism, Gram-negative sepsis, pancreatitis, leukemia.

Decreased Cholesterol. Hepatic diseases and insufficiency, Tangier disease, hyperthyroidism, β-lipoproteinemia, malabsorption and malnutrition, pernicious anemia, hemolytic jaundice, neurologic disorders, including epilepsy, Gaucher's disease, uremia, acute infection and sepsis.

Elevated Calcium. Since some of the calcium is bound to plasma protein, especially albumin, the determination of plasma albumin concentration is necessary before the significance of the calcium concentration result can be interpreted. The calcium concentration is regulated by endocrine, renal, gastrointestinal, nutritional factors, disorders of acidosis, primary and secondary hyperparathyroidism, hypervitaminosis D, early chronic renal failure, milk-alkali syndrome, hyperthyroidism, sarcoidosis, multiple myeloma, leukemia, prolonged immobilization, carcinoma of the lung and kidney, neoplastic bone involvement (osteolytic malignancy, lymphoma, secondary bone carcinomatosis).

Decreased Calcium. Hypoparathyroidism, pseudohypoparathyroidism, pseudopseudohypoparathyroidism, hypovitaminosis D (rickets, osteomalacia), tetany, blood transfusion reaction, late chronic renal failure, renal tubular acidosis, acute pancreatitis, malnutrition and malabsorption syndrome (steatorrhea, sprue, celiac

Table 2.4
SMA₁₂ Serum Analysis

Determinations		Normal Range
Calcium		9.0–11.0 mg%
Phosphorus	adult	3.0–4.5 mg%
	children	4.0–6.5 mg%
Glucose	2hr postprandial	70.0–110.0 mg%
	Folin-Wu 90–140.0 mg%; Somogyi-Nelson:	80.0–120.0 mg%
BUN (amino acids)		10.0–23.0 mg%
Uric acid (nucleoprotein)		2.5–8.0 mg%
Cholesterol		120.0–260.0 mg%
Total protein		6.0–8.0 gm%
Albumin		4.0–5.5 gm%
Total bilirubin		0.2–1.5 mg%
Alkaline Phosphatase		
International units		30–105
Bodansky units		1.5–4.5
King-Armstrong units		4–13
LDH ⎫ tissue destruction		100.0–225.0 IU/ml
SGOT ⎭		8.0–45.0 IU/ml

Note: Consult the laboratory for their normal values.
Other:

NA	136–145 mEq/liter	
K	3.5–5.5 mEq/liter	
Cl	98–106 mEq/liter	SMA₆ Serum analysis
CO₂	22–30 mEq/liter	
	Glucose and BUN	
1 minute (direct) bilirubin	0.1–0.4 mg%	
Creatinine	0.6–1.3 mg%	

disease, ileitis, necrosis of the pancreas), alkalosis, hypoproteinemia.

Elevated Inorganic Phosphorus. Renal insufficiency, nephritis, uremia, hypervitaminosis D, hypoparathyroidism, diabetic ketoacidosis (metabolic acidosis), healing bone fracture, acromegaly, hemolysis.

Decreased Inorganic Phosphorus. Hyperparathyroidism; elevated serum calcium, ingestion of antacids, negative nitrogen balance, Fanconi syndrome, myxedema, hepatic disease, high carbohydrate (CHO) intake, insulin at high doses, osteomalacia.

Elevated Bilirubin. Indirect reacting (unconjugated, prehepatic) and direct reacting (conjugated, hepatic or posthepatic), destruction of the hemoglobin yields bilirubin which is conjugated in the liver to the diglucuronide and excreted in the bile. Disorders include hepatitis, alcoholic (Laënnec's) cirrhosis, liver injury, obstruction of the flow of the bile (hepatoma, liver metastasis, pancreatic cancer, cholelithiasis), infectious mononucleosis, hemolytic anemia, pernicious anemia, eclampsia, Gilbert's disease, syndromes (Grigler-Najjar, Dubin-Johnson), and physiologic disorders such as icterus neonatorum or erythroblastosis fetalis.

Elevated Albumin. Dehydration (diuretic, vomiting, diarrhea), shock, hemoconcentration.

Decreased Albumin. Hepatic disorders (acute or chronic insufficiency, cirrhosis), starvation, malnutrition and malabsorption, low protein intake, diarrhea, cachexia, leukemia and other neoplastic diseases, systemic lupus erythematosis, nephrosis and nephrotic syndrome (diabetic glomerulosclerosis, glomerulonephritis), severe burns, exfoliative dermatitis.

Elevated Total Protein. Acute liver disease, cirrhosis of the liver, overwhelming acute and chronic infections, dehydration malnutrition, dysproteinemia, hypersensitivity condition, sarcoidosis, rheumatoid arthritis, multiple myeloma and other malignant neoplasms.

Decreased Total Protein. Compromised liver function, inadequate protein intake, metabolic disorders, starvation, malnutrition, malabsorption, cachexia, anemia, lymphatic leukemia, acute nephritis, nephrosis, edema, alcoholism, granulomatous diseases.

Elevated Uric Acid. Increased nucleoprotein catabolism, decreased renal excretion. Uric acid, an end product of nucleoprotein metabolism, is excreted by the kidney. It is elevated in primary gout, renal failure, thiazide diuretics, salicylates, ETOH abuse, plumbism, antineoplastic chemotherapy, toxemia (eclampsia) of pregnancy, starvation, Lesch—Nyhan syndrome, glycogen storage disease, anemia (hemolytic, pernicious), psoriasis, polycythemia, infectious mononucleosis, myeloproliferative diseases of the bone marrow (leukemia, lymphoma).

Decreased Uric Acid. Acute hepatitis, allopurinol, probenecid.

Elevated BUN. Urea, an end product of protein metabolism, is excreted by the kidney. Its concentration varies directly with protein intake and indirectly with the rate of excretion of the urea. It increases in glomerulonephritis, renal failure, pyelonephritis, glomerulosclerosis, renal calculi (obstructive uropathy), decreased renal blood flow, renal tuberculosis, renal neoplasm, high protein intake, severe protein catabolism (fever, extensive trauma, burn, severe infection), gastrointestinal bleeding, dehydration.

Decreased BUN. Cirrhosis of the liver, hepatic failure, cachexia (terminal cancer), amyloidosis, starvation, malabsorption, inadequate protein intake (negative nitrogen balance), nephrosis, and in pregnancy.

Elevated Glucose. Diabetes mellitus, stress, Cushing's disease and syndrome (adrenocortical hyperactivity, corticosteroid therapy), nephrosis, pheochromocytoma, acromegaly (hyperpituitarism), hyperthyroidism, pancreatitis, pancreatectomy, glucagon secreting tumor of the alpha cells of the islets of the Langerhans, Fanconi's syndrome, increased intracranial pressure (subarachnoid hemorrhage, brain trauma, hypertensive crisis), sepsis, thiazide diuretic, nicotinic acid excess, congestive heart failure.

Decreased Glucose. Functional hypoglycemia, prediabetic hypoglycemia, starvation, insulinoma (insulin-producing tumor), mesenchymal neoplasm that consumes glucose, massive hepatic necrosis, Addison's disease (adrenal cortical insufficiency), myxedema, cretinism, hypothyroidism, hypopituitarism, bacterial sepsis, excess insulin, glycogen storage disease, neoplasms (carcinoma, sarcoma, fibroma), congenital adrenal hyperplasia.

Elevated LDH. LDH catalyzes the conversion of lactate and pyruvate in the presence of NADH-NADH$_2$. It is distributed in body cells and fluids, elevated in all conditions accompanied by tissue infarction and necrosis. Individual isoenzymes may be elevated depending on what tissues are involved, i.e., the heart (myocardial infarction), erythrocytes (hemolytic anemia), liver (hepatitis and liver diseases), striated muscle (skeletal muscle trauma, seizures, surgery), kidney (acute renal infarction), lung (pulmonary infarction), skin (injury). Furthermore sprue, excessive nicotinic acid intake, benign and malignant neoplasms (carcinoma, lymphoma, leukemia) can elevate the LDH.

Elevated Alkaline Phosphatase. Alkaline phosphatase is present in high concentrations in bone and bile. It is increased if hepatic excretion is impaired, in hyperparathyroidism, hyperthyroidism, cirrhosis, hepatitis, liver cancer, hepatobiliary disease (obstructive liver disease), increased osteoblastic activity (Paget's disease, healing bone fracture), rickets, osteomalacia. myositis ossificans, primary malignant bone neoplasms, metastatic carcinoma involving bones, sarcoidosis, Gaucher's disease, pregnancy, congestive heart failure.

Decreased Alkaline Phosphatase. Hypophosphatasia, hypophosphatasemia, malnutrition, magnesium deficiency, hypothyroidism, pernicious anemia.

Elevated SGOT. SGOT (SGPT) intracellular enzyme present in high concentrations in muscle, liver and brain. Its increase in the blood indicates hepatic necrosis, active cirrhosis, acute (viral, toxic) hepatitis, hepatic metastatic carcinoma, obstructive hepatobiliary disease, infectious mononucleosis with hepatitis, muscle trauma (convulsions, gangrene, surgery, strenuous exercise, muscular dystrophy), body irradiation, severe burns, dermatomyositis, acute myocardial infarction, pulmonary infarction, acute renal disease, renal infarction, acute pancreatitis, acute hemolytic anemia, alcoholic neuropathy, brain trauma or necrosis.

Decreased SGOT. Uncontrolled diabetes mellitus with acidosis, liver dysfunction, beriberi.

9. Blood Glucose

Capillary blood sugar: detection of hyperglycemia in diabetic dental patients is important since it may be directly related to complicated or delayed healing; unsatisfactory periodontal therapy; ulcers, granulomas, thrush are more frequent; severe systemic problems, e.g., cardiovascular, cerebral, renal.

Determination of blood sugar concentrations: in patient with mild diabetes, a fasting blood glucose may be normal, but postprandial blood glucose will be elevated.

The two-hour postprandial blood glucose estimation is the most useful in a dental office. Administer approximately 100 gm carbohydrate, or moderate breakfast. Use a Dextrostix reagent strip. The urine should also be tested for glucose parallel with this test.

The fasting blood sugar is recorded after overnight fasting (problematic since diabetic outpatients may not tolerate hypoglycemia without fainting). The GTT (glucose tolerance test) is used in cases of high suspicion of diabetes mellitus on patients having a normal two-hour postprandial (four-hour) test. Measurement of the insulin reserve is the most exact diagnostic procedure.

Dextrostix procedure: apply capillary or venous blood to cover the entire reagent area on the strip (the reagent area must match "0" block on the chart, otherwise discard) following the fingertip or earlobe prick. Use only whole blood, do not squeeze the punctured area (connective tissue fluid). Wait 60 seconds. Wash for 2 seconds. Read immediately by using refractometer or visual reading (matching the color of the indicator with the chart on bottle). Note: chilled blood should be restored to room temperature before testing since the enzymatic reactions are depressed by temperature.

Indication: select out diabetics and suspected diabetics and measure the degree of control before dental procedures. Normal range of blood sugar is 70 to 100 mg% at fasting state; after intake of 100 gm CHO it rises to 160 mg% and returns to normal in two hours. Meal: slower absorption, Glucola: fast absorption. When the two-hour postprandial blood glucose level is above 120 mg% the patient may be prediabetic or an overt diabetic.

Whole venous blood values: Somogyi-Nelson: 80 to 120 mg%; Folin-Wu: 90 to 140 mg%; capillary blood values are approximately 30% higher than venous ones (arterial blood). Dextrostix has glucose oxidase and a color indicator system; between 40 and 250 mg% the error is 40%.

10. Urinalysis

The urine need not be clear, but should be well mixed. If blood glucose goes over 180 mg% (exceeding the renal threshold for glucose) it will spill into the urine (glucosuria). Most uncontrolled diabetics will therefore give a positive test for urinary sugar following a meal.

Combistix	Bili-Labstix
Glucose	Protein
Protein	pH
pH	Ketones
	Bilirubin
	Hemat
	Glucose

Procedure:
a. Collect morning urine in a clean container.
b. Dip the test portion of the strip (remove excess urine by touching the tip against the container).
c. Wait 10 seconds.
d. Do not wash.
e. Compare the midportion of the emulsion surface of the strip with the glucose color chart (qualitative test, i.e., the intensity of color change is not directly related to the glucose concentration).

Renal glucosuria: stress (glucocorticoids, epinephrine); normal blood sugar; renal disease; hyperglycemia (increased glucagon, anterior pituitary, thyroid); positive in 10% of pregnancies; inhibited tubular reabsorption (heredity); MI; GI infection; sepsis; increased intracranial pressure; ingestion of extra high carbohydrate meal.

Acetonuria (and diacetic acid—also called ketone bodies): clinically both acetone and acetoacetic acid have the same significance; may be detected in starvation, diabetic acidosis, pregnancy, dehydration, by using Ketostix, or Acetest tablets (sensitive as low as 5 mg% urine). The normal urine is negative for ketones.

Proteinuria (albuminuria): approximately 100 mg/24 hr (1500 ml) urine is normal. Functional: vascular, exercise, cold, pregnancy, orthostatic; pathologic: renal diseases. Note: the time factor after dipping is not critical for protein.

Hematuria: tumors, nephritis, nephrolithiasis, blood dyscrasias, GU infections, GU strictures, drug toxicosis. False: during menstruation, exercise.

Color: Normal urine is pale yellow and quite clear. Milky: pus, chyluria. Red: drugs (phenolphthalein, Sulfonal, Pyramidon, picric acid; hematuria; hemoglobinuria (sickle cell crisis, paroxysmal nocturnal hemoglobinuria, acute severe hemolytic reaction, transfusion reaction); food pigments (beets). Green: jaundice (biliary obstruction, hepatitis); typhus; cholera. Brown: bile; acute febrile disease; GU hemorrhage; porphyria; methemoglobinuria; myoglobinuria; melanin; alkaptonuria (homogentisic acid, the urine darkens on standing); Pyridium.

Specific gravity (1.010 to 1.016; dilution-concentration).

Microscopy (sediment): casts, bacteria, parasites; cells (RBC, WBC, renal tubule cells); amorphous material, crystals.

11. Occult Blood in Stool

With a round wooden applicator a bit of stool is smeared on a clean slide or mix feces in a test tube containing 5 ml of water and add reagent:
a. Benzidine: green → blue → purple in 15 minutes.
b. Gum guaiac: blue color is a positive reaction.
c. Peroxide-orthotolidine (Hematest tablet, Hemastix dipsticks) blue color is a positive reaction.
d. They all detect "heme" pigment, or Hb after hemolysis (deep blue).

False positive: undigested meat; enzymes in ingested food (pale blue).

12. Smear for Light Microscopic Examination

Smears of exudates, sputum, etc., are easily made and examined in the dental office: microorganisms, e.g., *Candida albicans*, fusiforms, actinomycosis; exfoliative cytology, e.g., Tzank cells (primary herpes simplex, varicella, herpes zoster, pemphigus), suspected carcinoma; and lavage cytology.

The most simple technique is as follows:
a. Smear a scraping of the lesion on the slide.
b. Allow to air dry.
c. Stain with Giemsa or toluidine (or methylene) blue or Gram stain depending on the situation.

13. Microbiologic Culture

Microbiologic culture should be utilized as indicated. Specimens may represent fluids removed from intact vesicle (herpes simplex, ECHO viruses, reoviruses, adenoviruses), throat washing, gargle (influenza), swab of freshly collected salivary secretion (mumps, tuberculosis), scrapings from the suspected lesions (ulcer), stool sample, etc.

14. Biopsy

Histopathologic tissue study is used to support the clinical diagnosis, e.g., aspiration (or needle), punch, incisional or excisional. If the histopathologic result is incompatible with the clinical diagnosis, the biopsy should be repeated in order to arrive at a definitive diagnosis. Note: if cancer is suspected, there is no contraindication to a biopsy. Electrocoagulation should follow the biopsy (seal off the lymphatics and blood vessels).

15. Normal Hematologic Values and Alterations

It can be expected that the majority of healthy individuals (about 95%) will be within the normal range represented.

Hb (hemoglobin)

Male: 14–18 gm%
Female: 12–16 gm%
High—same as for RBC.
Low—same as for RBC.

Hct (hematocrit)

Male: 40–54%
Female: 37–47%
High—polycythemia and dehydration.
Low—anemia, chronic hemorrhage.
Note: the Hct in children is age related.
2 years: 35.5%
4 years: 37.1%
8 years: 38.9%
12 years: 39.6%

RBC

Male: $4.5-6.0 \times 10^6/mm^3$
Female: $4.0-5.5 \times 10^6/mm^3$
High—polycythemia, dehydration.
Low—anemias, chronic hemorrhage, increased erythrocyte destruction, bone marrow failure.

WBC

$4,000-11,000/mm^3$

Differential

Myeloblasts, promyelocytes, mylocytes	0	0%
Neutrophils		
Metamyelocytes	$0-100/mm^3$	0–1%
Bands	$0-500/mm^3$	0–5%
Segments	2,500–6,000/mm³	40–60%

Neutrophils:
High—myelogenous leukemia, acute infectious disease, erythroblastosis fetalis, intoxication by drugs and poisons.
Low—malignant neutropenia, aplastic anemia, lymphocytic leukemia.

Lymphocytes $1,000-4,000/mm^3$ 20–40%
High—mumps, German measles, whooping cough, chronic infections, convalescence from acute viral infections, lymphocytic leukemia.
Low—aplastic anemia, myelogenous leukemia.

Monocytes $200-800/mm^3$ 4–8%
High—infectious mononucleosis, Hodgkin's disease, Gaucher's disease, malaria, monocytic leukemia, tuberculosis, subacute bacterial endocarditis.
Low—aplastic anemia.

Eosinophils $50-300/mm^3$ 1–3%
High—allergic disease, scarlet fever, some dermatoses, protozoan diseases, trichinosis, eosinophilic leukemia.
Low—aplastic anemia, typhoid fever, cortisone therapy, stress.

Basophils $0-100/mm^3$ 0–1%

Reticulocytes 0.5–1.5%

Platelets 200,000–400,000/mm³

High (thrombocytosis) — hemolytic anemias, polycythemia vera, chronic myelocytic anemia, acute rheumatic fever.

Low (thrombocytopenia)—thrombocytopenic purpura, symptomatic purpura associated with chemical or physical agents, acute and chronic leukemias, pernicious anemia, hemolytic jaundice, Banti's disease, Gaucher's disease, infective endocarditis.

RBC Indices (Wintrobe)

MCV (Mean Corpuscular Volume)

$$(cu\mu) = \frac{Hematocrit}{RBC}$$

Normal   82–92 cuμ
Normocytic anemia 82–92 cuμ
Macrocytic anemia 95–150 cuμ
Microcytic anemia   50–80 cuμ

MCH (Mean Corpuscular Hemoglobin)

$$(\mu\mu) = \frac{Hemoglobin}{RBC}$$

Normal   27–31 μμg
Normocytic anemia 25–30 μμg
Macrocytic anemia 30–50 μμg
Microcytic anemia   15–25 μμg

MCHC (Mean Corpuscular Hemoglobin Concentration)

$$gm/100\ ml = \frac{Hemoglobin}{Hematocrit}$$

Normal   32–36 gm/100 ml
Normocytic anemia 32–36 gm/100 ml
Macrocytic anemia 32–36 gm/100 ml
Microcytic anemia   25–30 gm/100 ml

White Blood Count

High (leukocytosis)—polycythemia, acute and chronic infections, exercise, fear, pain, leukemia.

Low (leukopenia)—neutropenia, depression of bone marrow, aplastic anemia, allergy, toxic reactions to drugs, respiratory tract infections, certain viral infections, cirrhosis, collagen disease, measles, typhoid and paratyphoid fever, influenza.

Morphology (stained blood smear gives information about the appearance of red blood cells).

1. Hypochromic alterations in color are associated with the reduction in hemoglobin concentration, i.e., iron deficiency, thalassemia.

2. Macrocytic and microcytic refers to the size of the red cells, i.e., B_{12}, folate deficiency.

3. Anisocytosis, poikilocytosis and spherocytosis alterations in the shape of the red cells.

Laboratory Diagnostic Code

Index (Indications of diagnostic laboratory procedures in some disease states)

1 = microhematocrit
2 = bleeding time
3 = capillary fragility
4 = venipuncture
5 = clot retraction
6 = blood clotting
7 = erythrocyte sedimentation rate
8a = sequential multiple analysis-12
8b = sequential multiple analysis-6
9 = blood glucose
10 = urinalysis
11 = occult blood in stool
12 = smear for light microscopic examination
13 = microbiologic culture and/or animal inoculation
14 = biopsy
15 = normal hematologic values

Indications of Laboratory Procedures in Diseases Listed

Actinomycosis

12 and 13—pus, tonsillar exudate to demonstrate the actinomycosis.

Acute Hemolytic Anemia

1   —Decreased.
4   —Neutrophilic leukemoid reaction, reticulocytosis.
       Hemoglobin electrophoresis.
       Decreased serum or plasma haptoglobins (α_2-globulins) as demonstrated by electrophoresis.
       If autoantibodies or isoantibodies are present the direct Coombs test is positive.

Increased indirect (nonconjugated) serum bilirubin.
Studies of peripheral blood smear = RBC morphology.
Sickle cell preparation is positive in sickle cell hemolysis.
Leukopenia in case of paroxysmal nocturnal hemoglobinuria.

11   —Hematuria, hemoglobinuria.

Acute Hemorrhagic Anemia

1   —After a time lag (2 to 12 hours) following an acute bleeding episode there is a drop of hematocrit due to hemodilution.
4   —For a couple of days:
Anemia (normochromic, normocytic).
Thrombocytosis.
Reticulocytosis.
Polymorphonuclear leukocytosis.

Acute Leukemia (Acute Myelocytic Leukemia, Acute Lymphocytic Leukemia)

1   —Decreased.
2   —Prolonged.
4   —Anemia, thrombocytopenia, peripheral leukocytosis (rarely granulocytopenia), sometimes pancytopenia (aleukemic leukemia).
Shift toward immature forms (myelocytic or lymphocytic cells).
12   —Bone marrow.

Acute Myocardial Infarction

4   —Polymorphonuclear leukocytosis for 2 weeks.
Elevated creatinine phosphokinase (CPK).
7   —Elevated for one month.
8a   —Increased LDH during the first week, elevated SGOT for the first two days.

Acute Pancreatitis

4   —Elevated: amylase, lipase.
Leukocytosis.
8a   —Elevated: bilirubin, BUN, alkaline phosphatase, SGOT.
Depressed: calcium.
Transient hyperglycemia.
8b   —Depressed: potassium.

10   —Elevated urinary amylase and amylase clearance.
Glucosuria (as related to transient hyperglycemia).

Acute Renal Failure

1   —Decreased.
4   —Anemia, low PH, raised creatinine.
8b   —Elevated BUN, hyperkalemia, hyperphosphatemia, hypocalcemia.

Acute Thyroiditis (Acute Infectious Thyroiditis, Suppurative Thyroiditis)

4   —Leukocytosis.
7   —Elevated.
13   —Isolate the pathogenic microorganisms from the thyroid.
14   —Acinary degeneration and multinucleated giant cells.

Addison's Disease (Primary Adrenal Cortical Insufficiency)

4   —Mild anemia (normocytic, normochromic).
Relative lymphocytosis.
Neutropenia.
Measure the steroid secretory response to a standard dose (50 units) of ACTH (the plasma cortisol increase should be at least 30 μg% in normal).
8b   —Hyponatremia, hyperkalemia, hypochloremia.
10   —Urinary 17-OHCS, 17-ketogenic steroids (17-KGS) or 17-ketosteroid level.

Adult Hypopituitarism (e.g., Sheehan's syndrome)

1   —Slight decrease.
4   —Anemia.
Depressed serum protein bound iodine.
17-Ketosteroid response to ACTH.
Thyroid hormone response to TSH.
8b   —Hypoglycemia, hyponatremia.
10   —Decreased urinary 17-ketosteroids and corticosteroids.
Positive metopyrone (Metopirone) test by blocking the production of cortisone, therefore, elevated level of ACTH would be re-

leased and increased urinary 17-hydroxy corticosteroids measured.

Amebiasis

4 —Serology.
12 —Intestinal wall scrapings, stool, pus, skin lesions for *Entamoeba histolytica*.
13 —Stool.

Anemias

1 —Decreased.
4 —RBC count, hemoglobin, RBC morphology and reticulocyte count, RBC indices, WBC count, platelet count.
14 —Bone marrow aspiration.

Angioneurotic Edema

4 —Identify the presence of active C'1 esterase inhibitor.

Aplastic Anemia (Pancytopenia)

1 —Decreased.
2 —Prolonged.
3 —Positive.
4 —Anemia (normocytic, normo-chromic).
Absolute reticulocytopenia.
Absolute granulocytopenia.
Thrombocytopenia.
12 —Bone marrow.

Asthma (Acute Reversible Airway Obstruction)

4 —Polymorphonuclear leukocytosis, eosinophilia.
12 —Sputum (Charcot-Leyden crystals, eosinophils, curschmann's spirals).

Bacterial Arthritis

12, 13 —Joint fluid, blood, urine, sputum, cervical exudate.

Bacterial Infections

4 —Neutrophilic leukemoid reactions.
7 —Elevated.
12, 13 —Blood, urine, exudate, sputum prior to antibiotic therapy.
Antibiotic sensitivity.

Bacterial Meningitis

4 —Seroreactions.
8a —Glucose, BUN, elevated LDH, protein.
8b —Hyponatremia.
12, 13 —Peripheral blood, cerebrospinal fluid to demonstrate *Diplococcus pneumoniae*, *Neisseria meningitidis*, *Haemophilus influenzae*, etc., elevated CSF protein, decreased sugar.

Blastomycosis (North American)

12 —Pus (*Blastomyces dermatitidis*).
13 —Urine, blood, cerebrospinal fluid, bone marrow, sputum, biopsy material.
14 —Involved site.

Bronchiectasis

1 —Decreased.
4 —Anemia (microcytic), neutrophil leukocytosis.
7 —Elevated.

Burkitt's Lymphoma

12 —From the cut surface of the tumor.
14 —Tumor site, bone marrow.

Candidiasis (Candidosis, Moniliasis, Thrush)

12 —Scrapings of skin and mucosal surfaces, appendages for *Candida albicans*.
13 —Culture of CSF, blood and joint fluid.

Cholera (Asiatic Cholera)

4 —Serology.
12, 13 —Feces for the *Vibrio cholerae*.

Chronic Granulocytic (Myelocytic) Leukemia

4 —Anemia.
Mild reticulocytosis.
Leukocytosis with immature granulocytes, "shift to the left" (neutrophils, eosinophils, basophils).
12 —Myeloid hyperplasia of the bone marrow.

Chronic Infections and Chronic Systemic Diseases

1 —May be depressed.
4 —May show anemia (normo-chromic, normocytic).

Chronic Lymphocytic Leukemia

1 —Depressed.
4 —Anemia (normochromic, normo-cytic), absolute lymphocytosis, thrombocytopenia, neutrope-nia.
8a —Hypo- (gamma) globulinemia.
12 —Bone marrow.

Chronic Renal Failure

1 —Depressed.
2 —Prolonged.
4 —Anemia (normochromic or hypo-chromic).
8a —Triglycerides, creatinine.
    In terminal stage: elevated phos-phate, protein, uric acid, BUN, glucose, alkaline phosphatase, decreased calcium.
8b —In terminal stage: elevated so-dium, potassium, chloride, de-creased bicarbonate.

Classic Hemophilia (Factor VIII, IX Disorder)

6 —Prolonged.

Clostridial Myonecrosis (Gas Gangrene)

12, 13 —Wound.

Coccidioidomycosis (Valley Fever)

4 —Leukocytosis, eosinophilia.
7 —Elevated.
12, 13 —For *Coccidioides immitis*.
14 —Involved site.

Collagen Vascular Diseases

See systemic (disseminated) lupus erythe-matosus, polyarteritis nodosa (periarteritis nodosa), scleroderma (progressive sys-temic sclerosis).

Common Cold (Acute Coryza)

1 —Decreased.
4 —Mild leukopenia (initial), relative lymphocytosis and late leuko-cytosis.
7 —Raised.

Coxsackie and ECHO Virus Infections (Aseptic Meningitis, Acute Undifferen-tiated Respiratory or Nonrespiratory Ill-ness)

4 —Serology.
13 —Virus isolation.

Coxsackievirus

Group A (herpangina, hand-foot-and-mouth disease or vesicular stomatitis with exanthem, acute lymphonodular pharyn-gitis).

Group B (epidemic pleurodynia, or Bornholm disease, epidemic myalgia, or devil's grip, myocar-ditis, pericarditis, orchitis).
4 —Serologic testing.
13 —Virus isolation.

Cryptococcosis (European Blastomycosis, Torulosis)

4 —Serology.
12, 13 —CSF, sputum, blood, pus to dem-onstrate the *Cryptococcus neo-formans*.
14 —Involved site.

Cushing's Syndrome

1 —Elevated.
4 —Erythrocytosis, granulocytosis, lymphopenia, eosinophilia, ele-vated plasma cortisol concen-trations (> 15 μg%).
    Dexamethasone (Decadron) test—ACTH suppression and low-ered plasma cortisol level.
8b —Hyperglycemia, hypokalemia.
10 —17-Hydroxycorticosteroids in ex-cess of 10 mg per gm of creati-nine.
    Metopyrone (Metopirone) test—blocks the productions of corti-sone, increases ACTH secre-tion, therefore elevates urine 17-OHCS.

Delirium

4 —CBC, pH.

8a   —Calcium, glucose, BUN, creatinine.
8b   —Potassium, sodium.

Diabetes Mellitus

4   —Positive glucose tolerance test (GTT).
         Fasting blood sugar (FBS).
8a   —Hyperglycemia, hyperlipemia.
10   —Glucosuria, proteinuria, ketonuria.

Diphtheria

13   —Swab from the suspected site for *Corynebacterium diphtheriae*.

Disseminated (Miliary) Tuberculosis

4   —Monocytic leukemoid reactions.
13   —Bone marrow culture.

Disuse Osteoporosis

10   —Elevated urine calcium.

Drug Allergy

4   —Basophil degranulation, eosinophilic leukemoid reactions.

Endemic Goiter

10   —Reduced excretion of iodine in the urine (less than 30 μg/day).

Eosinophilic Granuloma

14   —Eosinophils, histiocytes.

Eosinophilic Leukemia

4   —Eosinophilia.

Felty's Syndrome

1   —Depressed.
4   —Anemia, neutropenia, thrombocytopenia, RF factors.

Fibrous Dysplasia

14   —site of the lesion.

Gastrointestinal Bleeding

1   —Decreased.
4   —Decreased hemoglobin, leukocytosis.
8   —Elevated BUN.
11   —Occult blood in stool.

Glomerulonephritis (Acute, Subacute, Chronic)

4   —Anemia (normochromic, normocytic).
         Slightly decreased hemoglobin, elevated creatinine.
7   —Moderately raised.
8a   —Hypoalbuminemia, hypercholesterolemia.
8b   —Hyperkalemia.
10   —Proteinuria, hematuria, casts = fatty, granular, RBC, hyaline and epithelial.

Gonococcal Disease

12   —Fluorescent antibody.
13   —Culture of *Neisseria gonorrhoeae*.

Heart Failure

8a   —Elevated bilirubin, hypoglycemia, elevated SGOT.

Hemolytic Anemia (Hereditary Spherocytosis, Hereditary Elliptocytosis, Enzyme Deficiencies, Immune Defects, Microangiopathy)

4   —RBC morphology, reticulocytosis, transient hemoglobinemia.
         Seroreactions to demonstrate antibodies.
8a   —Elevated serum bilirubin and LDH, decreased haptoglobin.
10   —Transient hemoglobinuria.

Hemophilus influenzae

12   —Suppuration, exudate, sputum.

Hepatic Disease (Viral Hepatitis, Chronic Liver Disease)

1   —Depressed.
4   —Anemia, granulocytopenia, thrombocytopenia.
         Hypoprothrombinemia.
6   —Prolonged (impaired hepatic synthesis of prothrombin, fibrinogen and factors V, VII, IX, X).
7   —Slight increase.
8a   —Hyperbilirubinemia, hypoproteinemia, hypoalbuminemia, hyper (gamma) globulinemia, hypoglycemia; elevated: alkaline phosphatase and SGOT (SGPT).

8b   —Hypokalemia.
10   —Pyuria, elevated urobilinogen and bilirubin, proteinuria, microscopic hematuria.

Hereditary Hemorrhagic Telangiectasia (Osler-Weber-Rendu Disease)

1   —Decreased.
4   —Iron deficiency anemia.

Herpes Zoster

4   —Serology.
12   —Scrapings from the base of an early vesicle.

Histoplasmosis

4   —Serodiagnosis.
12   —Ulcer, swab (*Histoplasma capsulatum*)
13   —Urine, sputum, blood, bone marrow, cerebrospinal fluid, lymph node material.

Hodgkin's Disease

1   —Slight decrease.
4   —Mild anemia, neutrophilic leukocytosis, thrombocytosis, mild eosinophilia.
Elevated leukocyte alkaline phosphatase activity
Elevated: serum α_2-globulin, fibrinogen, haptoglobin.
Decreased serum iron and iron binding capacity.
7   —Elevated.
8a   —Elevated alkaline phosphatase, hypercalcemia, hyperuricemia, hypergammaglobulinemia
10   —Increased hydroxyproline, muramidase (lysozyme).
12   —Reed-Sternberg cells in the peripheral blood.
14   —Lymphoid tissue, enlarged lymph nodes, bone marrow (aspiration or open surgical technique).

Hyperparathyroidism

1   —Depressed.
4   —Anemia, radioimmunoassay for PTH in the peripheral plasma.
7   —Elevated.
8a   —Hypercalcemia, hypophosphatemia.

8b   —Hyperchloremia, hypokalemia, low serum bicarbonate.
10   —Hypercalciuria, increased urinary cyclic 3'-5'-AMP (the normal ratio of cyclic AMP to creatinine in the urine is 2.7 μmoles per gram of creatinine).

Hyperpituitarism (Acromegaly)

4   —Plasma growth hormone radioimmunoassay assessment.
Pseudodiabetic GTT.
10   —Elevated hydroxyproline level, glycosuria, hypercalciuria.

Hypersplenism

1   —Depressed
4   —Anemia.
Peripheral blood cytopenia (pancytopenia), including thrombocytopenia.
14   —Bone marrow: hypercellularity of normal elements.

Hyperthyroidism (Graves' or Basedow's Disease, Thyrotoxicosis)

4   —Mild anemia, hypokalemia.
Free thyroid hormone (FT_3 = triiodothyronine; FT_4 = thyroxine) index.
Radioactive iodine uptake (RAIU).
Slight increase in lymphocytes.
8a   —Increased serum calcium.
Elevated alkaline phosphatase.
10   —Increased calcium and hydroxyproline excretion.

Hypoparathyroidism

8a   —Hypocalcemia, hyperphosphatemia.
10   —Reduced urinary 3'-5'AMP.
Low urinary phosphate clearance.

Hyposplenism

12   —Peripheral blood for: Howell-Jolly bodies, nucleated red cells, target cell, siderocytes, Heinz bodies and acanthocytes.

Hypothyroidism and Myxedema

1   —Depressed.
4   —Anemia.

Elevated: CPK, TSH (> 20-1000 μu/cc).

Low: PBI, FT$_4$, RAIU.

8a   —Elevated: Cholesterol, LDH, SGOT.

CSF: elevated protein.

Infectious Mononucleosis (Pfeiffer's Glandular Fever)

4   —Elevated number of mononuclear leukocytes (lymphocytes, monocytes) may comprise 20–60% of the leukocytes, (lymphocytic leukemoid reactions).

Atypical lymphocytes.

Serologic evidence of both heterophil antibodies and cold reacting antibodies (Paul-Bunnel or presumptive test and differential absorption procedure, e.g., Monospot test and Mono-Test).

8a   —Elevated SGOT, SGPT and alkaline phosphatase.

10   —Hematuria.

Infectious Rhinitis

12   —Nasal smear (polymorphonuclear leukocytosis).

Infective Endocarditis (Bacterial Endocarditis, Prosthetic Valve Endocarditis)

1   —Decreased.

4   —Mild anemia (normochromic, normocytic) moderate leukocytosis, abnormal histiocytes.

10   —Proteinuria, microscopic hematuria.

13   —Blood culture (e.g., *Streptococcus viridans, Staphylococcus aureus*).

Influenza

4   —Serodiagnosis.

13   —Isolation of virus from sputum or throat washings.

Iron Deficiency Anemia

1   —Depressed.

4   —Anemia (microcytic, hypochromic), low serum iron concentration (normal: 175 μg%); increased total serum iron-binding capacity (normal: 410 μg%).

Thrombocytosis.

14   —Bone marrow: mild erythroid hyperplasia, low iron stores.

Klebsiella pneumoniae (Friedländer's Pneumonia)

4   —Leukocytosis (marked leukopenia marks grave prognosis).

13   —Blood, sputum.

Leukemoid Reactions

4   —Leukocytosis.

Leukopenia and Agranulocytosis

4   —Granulocytopenia.

14   —Bone marrow.

Lymphocytic and Histiocytic Lymphomas

4   —Lymphocytosis.

14   —Bone marrow, lymph nodes.

Macroglobulinemia (Waldenström's Macroglobulinemia)

1   —Decreased.

2   —Prolonged due to:

a. Interaction between IgM and coagulation factors.

b. Interference with platelet function (agglutination).

c. Capillary damage secondary to increased serum viscosity.

4   —Anemia, absolute lymphocytosis with "atypical, immature, and plasmacytic" forms.

7   —Elevated.

8a   —Elevated quantities of M-type (IgM) globulins.

12, 14 —Aspiration: peripheral blood, bone marrow, lymph node to demonstrate the proliferating lymphocytic-plasmacytic forms.

Malabsorption Syndrome

1   —Decreased.

4   —Anemia.

6   —Increased prothrombin time.

8a   —Decreased: calcium, albumin, cholesterol.

8b   —Decreased potassium.

Megaloblastic Anemia (B$_{12}$ and Folic Acid Deficiency)

1   —Lowered.

4   —Anemia (macro-ovalocytic), meg-

aloblasts in the buffy coat, thrombocytopenia, leukopenia with polymorphonuclear hypersegmentation.

8a   —Hyperbilirubinemia,   elevated LDH.

Meningococcal Disease

4   —Leukocytosis.
12   —*Neisseria meningitidis* from the buffy coat.
13   —Cerebrospinal fluid

Metastatic Diseases of the Bone Marrow

4   —Neutrophilic leukemoid reactions to pancytopenia.

Multiple Myeloma (Plasma Cell Myeloma, Myelomatosis)

1   —Depressed.
4   —Anemia (normochromic, normocytic).
      May have: leukopenia, thrombocytopenia (bleeding diathesis and interaction of M-type immunoglobulins and clotting factors).
      Relative lymphocytosis (40–55%).
      Plasma cells in the peripheral blood.
6   —Prolonged.
7   —Elevated.
8a   —30% may have hypercalcemia.
10   —M-type proteinuria, (Bence Jones) hyperuricosuria.
14   —Bone marrow (myeloma cell infiltration).

Mumps (Epidemic Parotitis)

4   —Leukocytosis, relative lymphocytosis, elevated serum amylase activity.
      Serodiagnosis.
13   —Isolation of the virus from saliva, urine, cerebrospinal fluid.

Mycoplasma (PPLO = Pleuropneumonia Like Organisms)

4   —Leukocytosis, neutrophilia, lymphopenia.
      Seroreactions.
7   —Elevated.

Myeloproliferative Disorder (Agnogenic Myeloid Metaplasia)

1   —Decreased.
4   —Anemia, (normochromic), leukocytosis (in 50%), leukopenia (in 25%).
      Reticulocytosis.
12   —Peripheral blood = immature granulocytes.
14   —Needle biopsy of the bone marrow (myelofibrosis or hypocellularity).

Neoplasms of the Esophagus (Esophageal Neoplasms)

12   —Lavage cytology.
14   —Biopsy.

Neoplasms of the Stomach (Gastric Neoplasms)

1   —Lowered.
4   —Anemia.
11   —Stool may be positive for occult blood.
12   —Exfoliative cytology.

Nephrotic Syndrome

8a   —Hypoalbuminemia,   hyperlipidemia (hypercholesterolemia).
10   —Proteinuria (over 3.5 gm/24 hours).

Nutritional Diseases

1   —Lowered.
4   —Hemoglobin.
8a   —Calcium, protein, albumin, cholesterol, BUN.
8b   —Potassium.

Osteitis Fibrosa

8a   —Hypercalcemia.
14   —Bone site involved.

Paget's Disease of Bone (Osteitis Deformans)

8a   —High serum alkaline phosphatase activity.
10   —Elevated urinary calcium excretion.

Paracoccidioidomycosis (South American Blastomycosis)

12   —*Paracoccidioides braziliensis.*

Parahemophilia (Factor V disorder)

6   —Increased prothrombin time.

Parasitic Involvement (e.g., Pneumocystis carinii in the saliva)

4   —Eosinophilic leukemoid reaction.

Pemphigus

12   —Skin and mucosal lesions.
14   —Soft tissue lesion.

Pertussis (Whooping Cough)

4   —Lymphocytic leukemoid reactions, leukocytosis.
13   —Nasal swab to isolate the *Bordetella*.

Pheochromocytoma

1   —Elevated.
4   —Polycythemia.
8a   —Hyperglycemia.
10   —Increased urinary excretion of free catecholamines (> 0-1 mg/24 hours), metanephrines (>1.3 mg/24 hours, normetanephrine, metanephrine), and vanillylmandelic acid (VMA, > 6.8 mg/24 hours).

Pneumococcal Pneumonia

4   —Leukocytosis (leukopenia in fulminating case).
      "Shift to the left" differential count.
13   —The sputum, blood, nasopharyngeal-tracheal aspirated material should be cultured for pneumococcus (*Streptococcus pneumoniae*).

Polycythemia

1   —Elevated.
4   —Reticulocytosis, leukocytosis, thrombocytosis, increased Hb.
8a   —Hyperbilirubinemia, elevated uric acid.
10   —Elevated urobilinogen.

Primary Aldosteronism (Conn's Syndrome)

4   —Decreased plasma renin (radioimmunoassay).

8b   —Hypokalemia, hypernatremia.
10   —High urinary aldosterone secretion rate.
      Normal 24 hour urine potassium (over 40 mEq/24 hours).

Pulmonary Embolism and Infarction

4   —Leukocytosis.
7   —Elevated
8a   —Increased bilirubin and LDH.

Purpura

2, 3 —Positive if there is no thrombocytopenia.
3   —Positive in case of hyperglobulinemia, senile nonhereditary type of vascular fragility, anaphylactoid, or allergic, pseudohemophilia or von Willebrand's disease (also positive no. 2, and abnormal platelet adhesiveness).
4   —CBC, platelet count.
      Decreased number or thrombocytopenia, may be secondary to hypersplenism (anemia, leukopenia), idiopathic thrombocytopenic purpura, bone marrow hyperplasia (aplastic anemia), replacement of marrow by fibrosis, neoplasm (like multiple myeloma), acquired immunologic thrombocytopenia (drug hypersensitivity reaction), B_{12} and folic acid deficiency (megaloblastic anemia), transfusion reaction.
      Increased number or thrombocythemia, e.g. chronic myelocytic leukemia, polycythemia vera.
12   —Bone marrow and peripheral blood smear.

Pyelonephritis

4   —Polymorphonuclear leukocytosis.
10   —White blood cell casts, red blood cells, pyuria, bacteriuria.
12   —Pus, urine sediment (bacteriuria).

Reiter's Syndrome

4   —Leukocytosis.

Respiratory Syncytial Virus Disease

4   —Leukocytosis.
     Serodiagnosis.
13   —Respiratory secretions.

Rheumatoid Arthritis

1   —Mild decrease.
     Moderate anemia, leukocytosis, eosinophilia, thrombocytosis, positive rheumatoid factors (RF; autoantibodies reactive with IgG), e.g., Plotz-Singer latex fixation tube test; Hyland RA test (latex slide test)
7   —Increased.

Rheumatic Fever

1   —Moderately decreased.
4   —Mild anemia, moderate leukocytosis, positive C reactive protein, serodiagnosis (antistreptolysin O titer > 200 Todd units).
7   —Elevated.
10   —Elevated RBC, WBC proteinuria.
13   —Throat culture (β hemolytic streptococci, Lancefield group A).
14   —Biopsy of subcutaneous nodules/Aschoff bodies (focal collagen necrosis surrounded by palisade arrangement of histiocytes).

Rickets and Osteomalacia due to Vitamin D Deficiency

8a   —Low phosphate, high alkaline phosphatase.
10   —Very low urine calcium.
14   —Bone (wide osteoid).

Rubeola (Measles, Morbilli)

4   —Serodiagnosis.
12   —Nasal exudate to demonstrate giant cells.
13   —Blood, urine, throat washings.

Sarcoidosis

4   —KMIF (Kveim-induced macrophage inhibition factor) tests the response of peripheral lymphocytes to macrophages.
     Leukopenia, eosinophilia.
8a   —Hypercalcemia, hyper(gamma) globulinemia, elevated alkaline phosphatase, hypoalbuminemia.
10   —Hypercalciuria, hydroxyprolinuria.
14   —Biopsy.

Scleroderma (Systemic Sclerosis)

1   —Mild depression.
4   —Moderate anemia, positive RF tests, presence of antinuclear antibodies (ANAs), LE cells, false positive serologic test for syphilis (STS).
7   —Elevated.
8a   —Mild hyper(gamma) globulinemia.
10   —Elevated urinary hydroxyproline.
14   —Skin, nodes.

Sickle Cell Anemia (Disease)

1   —Depressed.
4   —Anemia (hemolytic; nucleated RBCs, anisocytosis, target cells, sickled cells).
     Mild leukocytosis.
     Moderate thrombocytosis.
     Reticulocytosis.
     Hemoglobin electrophoresis.
8a   —Elevated bilirubin.
10   —Hematuria, hemoglobinuria.
14   —Bone, marrow (marked erythroid hyperplasia).

Sideropenic Dysphagia (Plummer-Vinson Syndrome, or Paterson-Brown-Kelly Syndrome)

1   —Decrease.
4   —Anemia (microcytic-hypochromic).

Sjögren's Syndrome

1   —Mild decrease.
4   —Mild anemia, RF factors, ANAs, LE cells.
7   —Elevated.
8a   —Hyperglobulinemia.
10   —Increased hydroxyproline excretion.
14   —Minor salivary glands (lymphoid infiltration).

Staphylococcal Pneumonia

4   —Leukocytosis.

13   —Sputum for Gram-positive cocci (located within polymorphonuclear leukocytes).

Streptococcal Sore Throat

4   —Serodiagnosis.
13   —Throat culture for group A, β hemolytic.

Stupor, Coma

4   —Complete blood count with differential.
8a   —Blood glucose, toxic substance screen, calcium, blood gases.
8b   —Sodium, potassium, bicarbonate.
10   —Toxic substance screen.

Subacute Thyroiditis (Granulomatous Thyroiditis, de Quervain's Thyroiditis)

1   —Depressed.
4   —Anemia, elevated T_4, PBI, depressed RAIU.
7   —Elevated.

Syphilis (Lues)

4   —Serologic tests (blood, cerebrospinal fluid), e.g., VDRL, TPI, FTA, FTA-ABS, TPHA.
12   —Lymph node aspirate, exudate from lesions for dark-field examination to demonstrate *Treponema pallidum*.

Systemic Lupus Erythematosus

1   —Moderate decrease.
2   —Mild increase.
4   —Moderate degree of anemia, leukopenia, thrombocytopenia, suppressed mononuclear leukocytes.
       Abnormal plasma proteins (cold-precipitating cryoglobulins, circulating anticoagulants, autoantibodies, elevated γ-globulins, "false positive" rheumatoid arthritis and serologic tests for syphilis).
       Positive LE cell preparation and fluorescent antinuclear antibody (ANA) test.
6   —Prolonged clotting, increased prothrombin time.
8a   —Hypoalbuminemia, hyperglobulinemia

10   —Microscopic hematuria, "telescoped" sediment (fatty-granular and RBC casts).

Tetany

8a   —Hypocalcemia.
8b   —Hypokalemia.

Thrombasthenia (Glanzmann's Disease)

2   —Prolonged.
5   —Reduced or absent.
6   —Increased.

Thrombocytopenia

1   —Decreased.
2   —Prolonged (purpura hemorrhagica, hemorrhagic diathesis).
4   —Thrombocytopenia, anemia. Seroreactions.
12   —Peripheral blood, bone marrow to see the megakaryocyte hyperplasia.

Thrombocytosis

2   —Prolonged.
4   —Thrombocythemia.
8b   —Pseudohyperkalemia (hyperkalemia due to release of potassium from platelets during blood clotting).

Toxoplasmosis

4   —Serology.
13   —Isolation of *Toxoplasma gondii* from sputum, blood, CSF or biopsy material.

Tuberculosis

1   —Decreased.
4   —Anemia (normocytic, normochromic).
8a   —Hyperglobulinemia, hypoalbuminemia.
8b   —Low serum sodium.
10   —Hematuria, pyuria (maybe).
12   —Sputum smear for *Mycobacterium tuberculosis*.
13   —Sputum, gastric aspirate, urine, bone marrow, cerebrospinal fluid, "deep cough."
14   —Suspected lesion.

Varicella

4   —Lymphocytic leukemoid reaction.

Vitamin D Resistant Rickets (Familial Hypophosphatemia)

8a   —Low plasma phosphorus.

High plasma alkaline phosphatase.

von Willebrand's Disease (Vascular Hemophilia)

2   —Long.
6   —Prolonged.

chapter

3

Dental Management of the Diagnosed, Medically Compromised Patient

JAMES V. MANZIONE

I. Introduction

Medical advances are allowing individuals to live longer lives and, as a result, dentists come in contact with a greater number of older patients who have underlying medical problems. In order to treat such medically comprised patients, the dentist must be cognizant of all medical problems by taking a detailed medical history. He must understand the significance of medical problems and how they affect his dental management of these patients.

Earlier chapters have already addressed the value and best way to detect and diagnose a patient's underlying medical problem. This chapter will concern itself with how the dentist must modify his dental management of patients based on their established medical profiles.

Each section of this chapter will discuss the types of medical problems commonly seen in the older adult patient, the likely medication he will be taking, and make certain recommendations regarding patient management in terms of procedure modifications, duration of visits, appropriate choice of drugs and anesthetics, drug interactions, need for oxygen, premedication, medical consultation and hospitalization.

At the outset, one should realize that the information in this chapter represents a set of guidelines and not a substitute for direct communication and consultation with the patient's physician. Consultations should be routine in all significantly compromised patients.

II. Cardiovascular Disorders

Cardiovascular disease affects a large portion of the American population and the dentist will deal with patients with these disorders daily. The cardiovascular disorders that the dentist will commonly encounter include angina, patient post-myocardial infarction, congestive heart failure, cardiac arrhythmias, hypertension, rheumatic fever and congenital heart disease.

a. Angina Pectoris

Angina should be suspected in any patient who experiences chest discomfort. Classically, angina is a retrosternal paroxysmal discomfort that may radiate to the arms, jaw, shoulders and back or may primarily be located in one of these areas. It typically feels like the pressure or sensation of a weight being applied to the chest. Anginal pain is normally of short duration, lasting minutes and brought on by exertion, emotional excitement, cold or eating.

Patients previously diagnosed as having angina can be taking any variety of medications. If angina occurs infrequently, a patient may only take sublingual nitroglycerin with each anginal episode. If angina

.occurs frequently in addition to p.r.n. nitroglycerin, a patient may also be taking oral or sublingual long-acting nitrates. Patients may also be taking propranolol, an agent that slows heart rate, decreasing oxygen requirements of the myocardium, thus decreasing myocardial ischemia and anginal attacks.

When the dentist suspects angina in a previously undiagnosed patient, medical consultation is required before any dental procedures, especially if the angina is of new onset or unstable, i.e., the nature of anginal episodes changes in terms of intensity, frequency or duration. New onset angina or unstable angina dictates complete medical evaluation since it may be the harbinger of acute myocardial infarction and, therefore, must be controlled before dental procedures are performed. Dental emergency procedures in patients with unstable angina should be undertaken in a hospital setting where appropriate medical backup is available to protect against the increased risk of acute myocardial infarction in these patients.

The patient with stable angina can be managed in the office setting after medical consultation regarding the severity of angina and the medications the patient is taking. When treating such patients, alleviating their anxiety and pain is most important. Satisfactory local anesthesia and mild sedation are also necessary. Allowing a patient to take nitroglycerin before performing a procedure or administering local anesthesia may prevent an anginal attack. Use of vasoconstrictors (i.e., epinephrine) in local anesthetic solution is not contraindicated in patients with mild, infrequent angina; however, its use should be avoided in patients with frequent angina because epinephrine will increase the heart rate and oxygen requirements of the myocardium and may precipitate an anginal attack. If the patient should develop angina during the dental procedure, nitroglycerin should be given. If pain persists, repeat nitroglycerin should be administered if the patient is not hypotensive, and the dental procedure should be terminated. Persistent pain may be secondary to an acute myocardial infarction and the patient should be transferrred to an emergency facility for evaluation. In patients with frequent angina, dental visits should be kept short. If the dentist anticipates extensive procedures or general anesthesia, then medical consultation and a hospital setting are required.

b. Postmyocardial Infarction

Many patients indicate a history of a myocardial infarction. In such patients the dentist ought to know when the infarction occurred and if it was complicated by congestive heart failure, cardiac arrhythmia or angina. It is generally agreed that only dental emergency procedures should be performed in patients who have had a myocardial infarction within the preceding three months. Medical consultation and a hospital setting are necessary for these patients, especially if a given patient experienced a complicated myocardial infarction. After six months, elective dental procedures can be performed in a stable patient. If the patient has angina, congestive heart failure or cardiac arrhythmia after a myocardial infarction, the precaution discussed under these headings should be considered. If the patient is three to six months status-post, a myocardial infarction medical consultation should be sought before doing elective or extensive dental procedures. No general anesthetics should be used in a nonhospital setting until six months after an infarction and should be performed only with medical consultation. Mild sedation and cautious use of epinephrine in local anesthetics is permissible in these patients. Vasoconstrictors in local anesthetics should be avoided if a patient has had myocardial infarction within the last three to six months and if a patient has had frequent angina and cardiac arrhythmias following an infarction.

Some patients following a myocardial infarction will be taking anticoagulants for a variable period of time. These patients are at an increased risk for bleeding and certain precautions should be taken as discussed in the hematology section of this chapter.

c. Congestive Heart Failure (CHF)

Congestive heart failure or cardiac insufficiency reflects an altered physiologic state of the left and/or right ventricle which may be the end result of a variety of conditions, i.e., hypertension, coronary artery disease, valvular heart disease, myocardiopathy, certain forms of congenital heart disease, thyroid disease, anemia or volume overload. Congestive heart failure is characterized by dyspnea on exertion. Other signs and symptoms that should raise the question of congestive heart failure in a patient are paroxysmal nocturnal dyspnea, tachycardia, orthopnea, cough to the extreme of pulmonary edema in left sided failure and ankle edema, distended neck veins and hepatomegaly in the case of right ventricular failure.

Patients with congestive heart failure will have restricted salt intake and be taking a diuretic and cardiac glycoside (digoxin or digitoxin). Most patients will have been previously diagnosed as having congestive heart failure when they see the dentist and, therefore, consultation with a patient's physician is necessary. If the dentist suspects that patients with CHF are poorly controlled or that CHF was previously undiagnosed as manifested by worsening or new onset of the above signs and symptoms, medical referral and consultation are needed to control maximally the patient's heart failure before dental procedures. Generally, patients who have only mild dyspnea with exercise can be treated in an office setting with appropriate use of mild sedation, avoidance of general anesthetics, short appointments and limited use of vasoconstrictors in local anesthetics, keeping the total epinephrine dose less than 0.1 mg. Patients with angina and cardiac arrhythmia associated with heart failure should have epinephrine eliminated in local anesthetics. Patients who experience dyspnea with less than normal exercise or dyspnea at rest should have only emergency dental procedures performed. These procedures should be performed with medical consultations in a hospital setting and with careful use of sedation, oxygen, diuretics, cardiac glycosides and limited use of epinephrine in local anesthetics, provided it is not contraindicated. General anesthetics should not be administered in patients with congestive heart failure without medical consultation and hospitalization.

d. Hypertension

Many physicians and scientists have offered opinions on hypertension over the years. Generally they agree that a patient is considered hypertensive if the systolic blood pressure is greater than 150 or the diastolic blood pressure is greater than 90. Many patients are unaware that they have hypertension and the dentist can play a major role in detecting hypertension by measuring the blood pressure of all patients. There is no doubt that treating hypertension decreases the death and complication rate of this disease and all patients found to be hypertensive should be referred to a physician for further evaluation and treatment prior to dental procedures. If a patient gives a history of hypertension, contact with his physician should be made to learn the extent of the patient's disease and degree of end organ involvement, i.e., nephropathy, retinopathy, cardiac involvement. A complete list of the patient's medications should be obtained and the possibility of any drug interactions between the drugs the dentist may use or prescribe and the various antihypertensive medications the patient may be taking should be evaluated.

Many of the antihypertensive agents today, especially reserpine, affect the sympathetic nervous system, thus orthostatic hypotension is a common problem. The patient's position should not be rapidly changed from the supine to the sitting or vertical position to avoid fainting or syncopal episodes.

Patients with well controlled hypertension can be treated in the office setting. It is best to avoid causing stress in these patients, therefore, short visits and mild sedation may be helpful. Pain control with local anesthetics also helps to avoid stressful situations. Epinephrine in local anesthetics may be used; however, total dose should be less than 0.1 mg.

In patients with poorly controlled hypertension, only emergency procedures should be performed and done so in a hospital setting due to the increased risk of bleeding, stroke and myocardial infarction in these patients. General anesthetics in any hypertensive patient require medical consultation and should be done in a hospital setting due to the risk of a hypotensive episode from a possible interaction of a general anesthetic with the various antihypertensive medications a patient may be taking.

e. Cardiac Arrhythmias

Cardiac arrhythmias are supraventricular (sinus bradycardia, sinus tachycardia, atrial premature contractions, supraventricular tachycardias, atrial flutter, atrial fibrillation) or ventricular (ventricular premature beat, ventricular flutter, tachycardia or fibrillation) in origin. Cardiac arrhythmias may be seen in association with any form of heart disease, i.e., hypertension, congestive heart failure, coronary artery disease. Generally ventricular arrhythmias are more life-threatening than supraventricular arrhythmias. The diagnosis and treatment of patients with arrhythmias requires extensive knowledge in this area and is beyond the scope of this discussion. Generally, when a patient presents to a dental office with a history of cardiac arrhythmia or if the dentist discovers an irregular pulse the patient's physician or cardiologist should be consulted regarding the type of arrhythmia the patient has, what medication he is taking and what possible drug interactions exist between the patient's antiarrhythmic medications and the drugs in the dentist's armamentarium. Patients with serious ventricular arrhythmias may require hospitalization for dental procedures, especially if extensive procedures or general anesthetics are required. When treating patients with arrhythmias, sedation is generally useful to decrease the release of endogenous catecholamines secondary to stress. Pain control is also important for the same reason. Local anesthetics should be used without vasoconstrictors since either exogenous or endogenous epinephrine can be arrhythmogenic in these patients.

In addition to drug therapy, some arrhythmias (bradycardia, sick sinus syndrome, complete heart block) require use of a pacemaker. Pacemakers either depolarize the heart at a fixed rate regardless of the underlying rate/rhythm of the heart or depolarize the myocardium only on demand when the intrinsic heart rate/rhythm is abnormal. Pacemaker function may be affected by electromagnetic radiation that may be produced by a variety of equipment in the dental office. When treating patients with pacemakers the patient's cardiologist should be consulted regarding which types of dental equipment or procedures may adversely affect pacemaker function. What is often not realized is that the pacemaker wire within the right ventricle is a foreign body similar to a prosthetic valve. Perhaps these patients need antibiotic premedication prior to dental manipulation. This point is controversial and should be discussed with the patient's cardiologist.

f. Rheumatic Heart Disease, Congenital Heart Disease and Other Cardiac Disorders Requiring Premedication with Antibiotics

Rheumatic fever primarily affects children and adolescents, although cases occur in young and middle-aged adults. It usually follows a group A β-hemolytic streptococcal pharyngitis and affects multiple organ systems. The diagnosis of rheumatic fever is established by satisfying the Jones criteria (five major and six minor criteria). To make the diagnosis of rheumatic fever one must fullfill two major or one major and two minor criteria. The major criteria include carditis, chorea, erythema marginatum, arthritis and subcutaneous nodules. The minor criteria include fever, elevated sedimentation rate, prolonged PR interval on ECG, history of rheumatic fever, and abdominal pain. The major concern in patients with a history of rheumatic fever is the presence of residual heart disease which predisposes the patient to infective endocarditis should bacteremia occur. Many patients with a history of rheumatic fever have no clinically apparent residual heart disease. These patients, however, may have subclinical abnormalities of the endocardium and it is, therefore, wise to provide antibiotic prophylaxis before dental procedures to all patients with a history of rheumatic fever. In addition to patients with a history of rheumatic fever, other patients at risk for infective endocarditis include most congenital heart disease, acquired valvular disease, idiopathic hypertrophic subaortic stenosis, mitral valve prolapse, indwelling transvenous cardiac pacemakers, dialysis patients with arteriovenous shunts and ventriculoatrial shunts in patients with hydrocephalus.

Patients at risk for infective endocarditis should maintain a high level of oral health since even in the absence of dental procedures periodontal disease and periapical infection may produce bacteremia. Oral ulcers from poorly fitting dentures can also cause bacteremia. In patients at risk for infective endocarditis antibiotic prophylaxis is recommended for all dental procedures that are likely to cause gingival bleeding. Devices that use water under pressure and dental flossing have been shown to cause bacteremia, however, bacterial endocarditis associated with the use of these has not been fully investigated. Caution is advised in their use by patients with cardiac defects, especially when oral health is poor.

Alpha hemolytic streptococci, (i.e., *Streptococcus viridans*) are the organisms most commonly found to cause bacterial endocarditis of dental origin and antibiotic prophylaxis should be directed towards them.

The most recent recommendations of the American Heart Association regarding antibiotic prophylaxis against infective endocarditis during dental procedures in susceptible patients are presented in Table 3.1 and 3.2.

Patients with prosthetic valves often are taking anticoagulants and they are at a greater risk for bleeding following dental and surgical procedures. The recommended precautions for patients taking anticoagulants are discussed in the hematology section of this chapter.

III. Pulmonary

a. Upper Respiratory Infections

In previously healthy patients, these infections are self-limiting. It is generally wise to postpone elective procedures until the upper respiratory infection has resolved, mainly to avoid exposure to the dentist and his staff. In addition, some patients with upper respiratory infections may have some difficulty breathing with the variety of dental apparatus placed in their mouths, i.e., rubber dam, cotton, etc. Emergency procedures can be performed without hesitation in previously healthy patients. It is recommended that the dentist and personnel treating such patients wear masks for their own protection.

b. Chronic Obstructive Pulmonary Disease (COPD)

The disorders included under this heading are asthma, chronic bronchitis and emphysema.

Asthma is a disorder characterized by reversible bronchospasm at times in response to an allergen, upper respiratory infection or other precipitating factors and is referred to as extrinsic asthma. Frequently no allergen or precipitating factor is identified and this is referred to as intrinsic asthma. The acute asthma attack is characterized by sudden onset of shortness of breath, dyspnea and wheezing. Its emergency treatment requires the attention of a physician and, should a patient present with an acute asthmatic attack, referral should be made without delay since extensive medical therapy and possibly hospitalization may be required. The management of asthma requires the use of various bronchodilators, including epinephrine (0.2 to 0.4 cc of 1:1000 solution subcutaneously), as soon as the diagnosis is made. In older patients with cardiovascular disease terbutaline subcutaneously should be used instead of epinephrine. In addition, various other bronchodilators are employed depending on the severity of the attack, i.e., bronchosol nebulizer, aminophylline and terbutaline. In more severe or refractory cases of bronchospasm, steroids and possibly intubation with hospitalization may be required. Some patients with asthma have a degree of chronic bronchospasm which should be optimally treated prior to dental procedures. Certain patients with asthma require chronic steroid therapy. These patients may need a pulse in their steroids when extensive dental procedures are anticipated since they may have adrenal suppression. Inhalation anesthetics should be avoided in patients with asthma since they may precipitate an

Table 3.1
Prophylaxis for Dental Procedures and Surgical Procedures of the Upper Respiratory Tract

	Most congenital heart disease;[c] rheumatic or other acquired valvular heart disease; idiopathic hypertrophic subaortic stenosis; mitral valve[d] prolapse syndrome with mitral insufficiency	Prosthetic heart valves[e]
All dental procedures that are likely to result in gingival bleeding[a, b]	Regimen A or B[g]	Regimen B
Surgery or instrumentation of the respiratory tract[f]	Regimen A or B	Regimen B

[a] Does not include shedding of deciduous teeth.

[b] Does not include simple adjustment of orthodontic appliances.

[c] For example, ventricular septal defect, tetralogy of Fallot, aortic stenosis, pulmonic stenosis, complex cyanotic heart disease, patent ductus arteriosus or systemic to pulmonary artery shunts. Does not include uncomplicated secundum atrial septal defect.

[d] Although cases of infective endocarditis in patients with mitral valve prolapse syndrome have been documented, the incidence appears to be relatively low and the necessity for prophylaxis in all of these patients has not yet been established.

[e] Some patients with a prosthetic heart valve in whom a high level of oral health is being maintained may be offered oral antibiotic prophylaxis for routine dental procedures except the following: parenteral antibiotics are recommended for patients with prosthetic valves who require extensive dental procedures, especially extractions, or oral or gingival surgical procedures.

[f] For example, tonsillectomy, adenoidectomy, bronchoscopy, and other surgical procedures of the upper respiratory tract involving disruption of the respiratory mucosa.

[g] See Table 3.2.

Table 3.1 is reprinted by permission of the American Heart Association from E. L. Kaplan, et al. Prevention of bacterial endocarditis, *Circulation*, 56:139A, 1977.

episode of bronchospasm. They should not be used without prior pulmonary function tests and consultation with a pulmonary physician or anesthesiologist. Good local anesthetics and mild non-narcotic sedation may be helpful in these patients to decrease the stress that may precipitate an acute asthma attack. Narcotics should be avoided since they cause release of histamine and may precipitate acute bronchospasm.

The dentist will frequently see patients with varying degrees of chronic bronchitis or emphysema usually secondary to chronic cigarette smoking. Chronic bronchitis is characterized by chronic sputum production, varying degrees of dyspnea on exertion, bronchospasm, and airway obstruction. All patients with bronchitis or suspected bronchitis should be referred to a physician for optimal treatment which often includes antibiotics, bronchodilators and chest physical therapy to correct bronchospasm and remove secretions. Inhalation anesthesia and narcotic sedation should be avoided in these patients due to the possibility of inducing bronchospasm. In patients with chronic bronchitis and COPD one should avoid use of high oxygen concentrations unless the capacity for measuring arterial blood gases is available. Many patients with significant obstructive airway disease either from severe asthma, bronchitis or emphysema have a blunted respiratory response to levels of PCO_2 in blood. These patients thus rely on their level of PO_2 to control the ventilatory drive. If oxygen is given indiscriminately to these patients they may suppress their PO_2 dependent ventilatory drive and thus decrease their effective alveolar ventilation, raise the PCO_2 and develop a respiratory acidosis. When these patients develop respiratory infections as manifested by increased cough, sputum production, dyspnea, shortness of breath and bronchospasm, dental procedures should be postponed, since these patients can develop a significant abnormality in gas exchange in association with respiratory infections. All patients with chronic bronchitis who have worsening symptoms or upper respiratory infections should be referred to a physician for optimal treatment prior to dental procedures.

In general, when confronted with patients with a history of asthma, bronchitis and emphysema, medical consultation

Table 3.2
Regimens for Dental Procedures and Surgery of the Upper Respiratory Tract

Regimen A—Penicillin	Regimen B—Penicillin plus Streptomycin
1. Parenteral-oral combined:	*Adults:* Aqueous crystalline penicillin G (1,000,000 units intramuscularly) *mixed with* procaine penicillin G (600,000 units intramuscularly) *plus* streptomycin (1 gm intramuscularly). Give 30 min to 1 hr prior to the procedure; then penicillin V 500 mg orally every 6 hr for 8 doses[a]
Adults: Aqueous crystalline penicillin G (1,000,000 units intramuscularly) *mixed with* procaine penicillin G (600,000 units intramuscularly). Give *30 min to 1 hr prior to procedure* and then given penicillin V (formerly called phenoxymethyl penicillin) 500 mg orally *every 6 hr for 8 doses*[a]	
Children:[b] Aqueous crystalline penicillin G (30,000 units/kg intramuscularly) *mixed with* procaine penicillin G (600,000 units intramuscularly). Timing of doses for children is the same as for adults. For children less than 60 lb the dose of penicillin V is 250 mg orally every 6 hr for 8 doses[a]	*Children:*[b] Aqueous crystalline penicillin G (30,000 units/kg intramuscularly) *mixed with* procaine penicillin G (600,000 units intramuscularly) *plus* streptomycin (20 mg/kg intramuscularly). Timing of doses for children is the same as for adults. For children less than 60 lb the recommended oral dose of penicillin V is 250 mg every 6 hr for 8 doses.[a]
2. Oral:[c]	*For Patients Allergic to Penicillin:*
Adults: Penicillin V (2.0 gm orally 30 min to 1 hr prior to the procedure and then 500 mg orally every 6 hr for 8 doses)[a]	*Adults:* Vancomycin (1 gm intravenously over 30 min to 1 hr). Start initial vancomycin infusion ½ to 1 hr prior to procedure; then erythromycin 500 mg orally every 6 hr for 8 doses[a]
Children:[b] Penicillin V (2.0 gm orally 30 minutes to 1 hour prior to procedure and then 500 mg orally every 6 hr for 8 doses.[a] For children less than 60 lb use 1.0 gm orally 30 min to 1 hr prior to the procedure and then 250 mg orally every 6 hr for 8 doses)[a]	*Children:*[b] Vancomycin (20 mg/kg intravenously over 30 min to 1 hr).[d] Timing of doses for children is the same as for adults. Erythromycin dose is 10 mg/kg every 6 hr for 8 doses[a]
For Patients Allergic to Penicillin:	
Use either vancomycin (see Regimen B) or use:	
Adults: Erythromycin (1.0 gm orally 1½–2 hr prior to the procedure and then 500 mg orally every 6 hr for 8 doses)[a]	
Children: Erythromycin (20 mg/kg orally 1½–2 hr prior to the procedure and then 10 mg/kg every 6 hr for 8 doses)[a]	

[a] In unusual circumstances or in the case of delayed healing, it may be prudent to provide additional doses of antibiotics even though available data suggest that bacteremia rarely persists longer than 15 min after the procedure. The physician or dentist may also choose to use the parenteral route of administration for all of the doses in selected situations.

[b] Doses for children should not exceed recommendations for adults for a single dose or for a 24-hr period.

[c] For those patients receiving continuous oral penicillin for secondary prevention of rheumatic fever, α-hemolytic streptococci which are relatively resistant to penicillin are occasionally found in the oral cavity. While it is likely that the doses of penicillin recommended in Regimen A are sufficient to control these organisms, the physician or dentist may choose one of the suggestions in Regimen B or may choose oral erythromycin.

[d] For vancomycin the total dose for children should not exceed 44 mg/kg/24 hr.

Table 3.2 is reprinted by permission of the American Heart Association from E. L. Kaplan, et al. Prevention of bacterial endocarditis, *Circulation*, 56:139A, 1977.

should be obtained to learn how much obstructive airway disease is present based on pulmonary function tests. If, based on these tests, obstruction is mild to moderate and a patient is under good control and maximal medical treatment, most dental procedures can be performed in the office setting, but inhalation anesthesia and narcotic analgesics should be avoided. In patients with marked chronic obstructive pulmonary disease, a hospital setting may be desirable.

IV. Central Nervous System

a. Strokes

Cerebrovascular disease is the most common of all neurological disorders. The term stroke refers to any pathologic process affecting the vessels of the brain such as thrombosis, embolism, rupture, etc. Cerebral deficits from strokes may be transient with full resolution of function within 24 hours as in transient ischemic attacks (TIA) or permanent when some residual deficit persists. A transient ischemic attack should be suspected in any patient who gives a history of transient paresthesias, dysesthesias, weakness, aphasia, etc. Patients with diabetes and high blood pressure are at an increased risk for developing TIA's and strokes. Patients who have suffered a TIA or stroke within the last six months should have their neurologist and internist consulted prior to dental procedures and only emergency procedures should be performed within this time period. Beyond six months in a stroke patient, it is generally safe to perform routine dental procedures following consultation with the patient's neurologist since certain precautions may need to be taken.

Following a stroke, depending on its nature, a patient may be taking an anticoagulant, which must be considered and is discussed in the hematology section of this chapter, when dental procedures are anticipated to avoid bleeding problems. In patients with a history of a TIA or stroke, sedation must be used very cautiously since a sudden fall in blood pressure may cause a worsening of the initial deficit or a new one. If general anesthesia is considered in these patients, it should be used in a hospital setting following consultation with a neurologist and anesthesiologist. Patients with high blood pressure should have their hypertension controlled prior to dental procedures. Dental visits should be short and well planned. Patients who have seizure disorders following a stroke need additional precautions taken, as discussed below.

b. Seizures

Approximately 0.5% of the population has some form of seizure disorder; in the majority of cases no underlying cause can be found. Generally, however, new onset of seizures in the adult is due to some form of organic disease.

There are four major types of seizure (grand mal, petit mal, Jacksonian and psychomotor) classified on the basis of seizure characteristics. For details concerning the manifestations and treatment of each type

of seizure reference should be made to any neurologic or general medical text.

If a patient has a history of a seizure disorder, the patient's physician or neurologist should be contacted regarding the patient's medication and degree of seizure control. Generally, there is no contraindication to dental therapy as long as the patient is taking his medication. If there is any question of a patient not complying with his medications, serum levels of most anticonvulsants are available. It is useful to plan visits at times when a patient's medication levels are at their peak. Generally, barbiturate premedication is useful, although not necessary in patients with well controlled seizures. Local anesthetics and vasoconstrictors are not contraindicated since these catecholamines do not cross the blood brain barrier. It is well known that gingival hypertrophy occurs with prolonged dilantin therapy. This may be minimized with good oral hygiene.

V. Gastrointestinal

a. Peptic Ulcer Disease

Many patients with peptic ulcer disease (duodenal ulcer and gastric ulcer) will be seen by the dentist. There are a few precautions the dentist may have to take when treating these patients. These patients may be taking a variety of medications and there are various medications that should be avoided in these patients. The main mode of treatment in these patients is to decrease gastric acid secretion. Antacids are the main mode of therapy. These drugs bind tetracycline and erythromycin and decrease their absorption, if these medications are given within one hour of antacids. Recently cimetidine, an H2 histamine receptor antagonist that decreases gastric acid secretion, has been introduced. This drug is similar to other H2 histamine receptor antagonists such as Metiamide, and like this drug may cause bone marrow suppression. Also, patients with peptic ulcer disease can slowly lose blood in the stool (melena or occult blood loss). Thus if surgical procedures are anticipated in patients with peptic ulcer disease, a complete blood count and platelet count should be done to determine if any blood loss or bone marrow suppression has occurred. Drugs that should be avoided in patients with peptic ulcer disease because of their ulcer-producing tendency are preparations containing aspirin, indomethacin, phenylbutazone or steroids.

b. Liver Disease

There are multiple forms of liver disease, i.e., cirrhosis, alcoholic or viral hepatitis, to mention a few. With extensive liver disease, either secondary to acute insult or chronic liver disease, abnormalities in the various metabolic and synthetic function of the liver may occur. With liver failure, there is inadequate synthesis of clotting factors and bleeding problems may occur. There is also decreased metabolism of ammonia and various drugs, including certain sedatives (barbiturates), predisposing these patients to metabolic encephalopathy.

Sedatives can be very dangerous in these patients and should be used with extreme caution and only following medical consultation since these patients may be exquisitely sensitive to them. In patients with a history of liver disease or in patients where liver disease is suspected, i.e., patients with jaundice, palmar erythema, spider angiomas, gynecomastia, etc., one should consult the patient's physician regarding the extent of the patient's liver disease in terms of synthetic and metabolic function and if any precautions need to be taken. Patients with significant liver disease with compromised metabolic or synthetic function should be treated in a hospital setting. Knowing the cause of a patient's liver disease is important. For example, if a patient is an alcoholic there are a number of other concerns aside from the patient's liver disease. These patients are malnourished and susceptible to blood loss from the gastrointestinal tract, secondary to either peptic ulcer disease, gastritis or varices. Thus a CBC and stool test for occult blood should be performed.

Viral hepatitis is of concern to the dentist since it is transmissible from patient to patient or patient to dentist during the prodrome or acute phase of the disease. Gloves should be used for all surgical procedures and proper sterilization procedures carried out as discussed in chapter five.

c. Malabsorption

There are a number of disorders that can cause malabsorption, namely, chronic pancreatic insufficiency, biliary tract disease, intrinsic bowel disease, etc. Many of these patients are malnourished and may be anemic. Synthetic liver function may be abnormal and abnormalities in clotting function may occur. Patients with malabsorption require medical consultation and CBC, especially if surgical procedures are anticipated.

d. Inflammatory Bowel Disease

Patients with inflammatory bowel disease such as Crohn's disease and ulcerative colitis are of concern to the dentist since they may be anemic from chronic gastrointestinal blood loss or chronic disease. These patients may also be taking steroids or immunosuppressive agents with their inherent problems discussed elsewhere in this chapter. Complete blood counts and medical consultations regarding the patient's medication and extent of the disease are indicated in these patients.

VI. Renal Disease

There are a large variety of renal diseases that a dentist may encounter. In any patient who gives a history of renal disease his internist or nephrologist must be consulted regarding the extent of this renal disease and precautions that need to be considered at the time of dental procedures. Patients with significant renal disease can have a variety of extrarenal complications. Cardiovascular complications include congestive heart failure, hypertension, edema and pericarditis. Gastrointestinal manifestations may consist of oral ulcers, parotitis, anorexia, hiccups, nausea, vomiting, mucosal ulceration, abdominal pain or pancreatitis. Hematologic abnormalities include normochromic normocytic anemia and a bleeding tendency resulting from capillary fragility, thrombocytopenia and/or poor platelet function. There is an unusual susceptibility to infection due to depression of leukocyte count and depression of cellular immunity. Mental clouding and lethargy are common as well as itching of the skin. Each of these complications must be considered by the dentist and the appropriate precautions taken which have been discussed in the various portions of this chapter. Patients with chronic renal failure will be getting dialysis, usually hemodialysis, and will have arteriovenous shunts or fistulas. These patients will generally need antibiotic premedications with dental procedures. The dosage of antibiotics in renal failure patients should be discussed with the patient's nephrologist, since the renal clearance of these drugs is absent or severely decreased and drug dosages may need to be altered. Patients with renal transplants will be taking steroid and immunosuppressive agents and appropriate precautions must be taken in these patients, as will be discussed later in this chapter.

VII. Endocrinologic Disorders

a. Diabetes

Diabetes mellitus occurs in a juvenile or adult onset form. Juvenile onset diabetics require insulin therapy, are more difficult to manage and are more likely to develop hypoglycemia, hyperglycemia or ketoacidosis than the adult onset diabetics. Adult onset diabetes may be controlled by diet alone but at times insulin or oral agents are also required. These patients are more easily managed and are less likely to develop wide swings in serum glucose or ketoacidosis. The symptoms of uncontrolled diabetes are polyuria, polydipsia and polyphagia. The long-term manifestations of diabetes include retinopathy with impairment of vision, nephropathy with impairment of renal function, peripheral neuropathy, vascular insufficiency with increased susceptibility to ulcer and infection of distal extremities, especially feet and toes, increased susceptibility to cardiovascular and cerebrovascular disease, increased susceptibility to infection, especially with candida. There are a number of

tests that are helpful in the diagnosis of diabetes. Testing for glycosuria is simple but both nonspecific and insensitive. Measuring the fasting blood glucose is a more specific test and determining the two-hour postprandial glucose level is a more sensitive test. The glucose tolerance test, however, is more likely to detect diabetes than either of the above tests and is the test generally used. Any patient who, gives a history of diabetes or the diagnosis, is suspected should have their physician consulted for either diagnostic purposes and treatment in the case of the suspected diabetic or for assessment of control, extent of end organ damage and need for precaution in previously known diabetics.

When treating diabetes, hypoglycemia is more of a concern than hyperglycemia. Often after a dental procedure a patient may not be able to eat, which will decrease his insulin requirement. If such a patient took his usual morning insulin dose there is a possibility that he may become hypoglycemic as manifested by tachycardia, diaphoresis, lightheadedness, syncope or even coma if severe hypoglycemia occurs. If it is anticipated that a patient's oral intake will be significantly decreased following a dental procedure, to prevent hypoglycemia, it is advisable that the patient decrease his morning insulin dose the day of the procedure. The exact modification of the patient's insulin dose will depend on the severity of the patient's diabetes and should be decided upon with the patient's physician if one is not experienced in treating diabetics. In very extensive procedures where a patient may have a prolonged decrease in oral intake or in patients with brittle diabetes a hospital setting where blood glucose can be monitored and controlled is necessary. Another consideration in diabetic patients is their susceptibility to infection. For simple procedures rarely is this a problem. However, for extensive surgical procedures or where infection exists, antibiotic coverage is advisable. Infection in diabetics can result in loss of control and predispose a patient to hyperglycemia or ketoacidosis, especially in the juvenile onset diabetic. In any diabetic with a significant infection, the patient should be questioned regarding symptoms of loss of diabetic control, i.e., polyuria, polydipsia, polyphagia, fatigue, weakness, increased respiratory rate, nausea, vomiting or abdominal pain. These patients should have their urine and serum tested for glucose since hyperglycemia and ketoacidosis may present insidiously in these patients and the diagnosis may not be suspected until the patient is critically ill.

Diabetics are also prone to hemorrhage due to their vascular disease and good hemostasis should be provided.

b. Thyroid Disease

Patients with hyperthyroidism have a variety of symptoms and metabolic abnormalities which may include any of the following: weight loss, nervousness, tremor, lid lag, exophthalmos, hair changes, gastrointestinal symptoms, heat intolerance, palpitations, tachycardia or hypertension. The diagnosis is confirmed by thyroid function test; the most widely used today are the radioimmunoassays for T_4, T_3 and T_3 resin uptake. Treatment consists of surgical or radiation ablation of the thyroid or medical management. Patients following radiation may require thyroid replacement. Medical management consists of antithyroid medication such as propylthiouracil which may produce bone marrow suppression or agranulocytosis.

If the dentist suspects hyperthyroidism in a patient, medical referral is indicated for appropriate thyroid function tests, thyroid scans and treatment, if needed. Dental procedures should be avoided in any patient suspected of or known to be hyperthyroid until the diagnosis is confirmed and the disorder controlled in suspected patients and the level of control is determined in previously diagnosed patients. This is important to prevent precipitating thyroid storm in untreated or poorly controlled patients with hyperthyroidism which may be life-threatening. Patients with hyperthyroidism are susceptible to cardiac irritability and epinephrine in local anesthetics is therefore contraindicated. Pain control as well as short visits and appropriate use of sedative premedication is important in these patients. Hypothyroidism is due to decreased function of the thyroid gland. Its diagnosis should be sus-

pected in any patient who has lethargy, cold intolerance, constipation, menorrhagia, weight gain, decreased appetite, dry hair that tends to fall out, congestive heart failure, cardiomegaly, deepening voice, or rough, dry skin. Patients with hypothyroidism receive thyroid replacement either in the form of a synthetic hormone or thyroprotein derived from animal thyroid. In patients suspected of being hypothyroid, medical referral is needed for appropriate thyroid function tests and treatment. Patients with known hypothyroidism should have their physician consulted regarding their level of control and the need for any precautions at the time of dental treatment. Factors that can precipitate myxedema coma in these patients include trauma, infection and central nervous system depressants. The dentist must keep this in mind when called to treat trauma or significant infection in these patients. Sedation should be avoided in these patients.

c. Adrenal Disease

Hyperfunction of the adrenal cortex known as Cushing's syndrome is characterized by truncal obesity, hypertension, edema, glycosuria, osteoporosis, amenorrhea, hirsutism, weakness, "moon" facies, abdominal striae, "buffalo" hump. There are many causes of Cushing's syndrome but each results in increased production of cortisol by the adrenal cortex. The treatment of Cushing's syndrome depends on its underlying cause, the details of which will not be discussed.

Treatment usually involves ablation of the adrenal glands through surgery or drugs. These patients then are subsequently treated with maintenance glucocorticoids. Patients with hypocorticism or Addison's disease are at the other end of the spectrum from patients with Cushing's syndrome. It is characterized by weight loss, weakness, hypotension, loss of appetite, vomiting, diarrhea, brownish pigmentation of the skin and mucous membranes, memory changes and headaches. The treatment of Addison's disease requires steroid replacement. In any patient in whom a history of or the diagnosis of hypercorticism or hypocorticism is suspected medical consultation is required for confirmation and control of the disorder or assessment of degree of control in previously diagnosed patients before any dental treatment is performed.

Adrenal hypofunction as in Addison's disease can result from a variety of causes, for example, patients treated for hypercorticism by surgery or durgs have resultant hypocorticism and as discussed above receive subsequent corticosteroid replacement therapy. Patients who take long-term steroids for any of a variety of reasons (usually collagen vascular or autoimmune diseases) will have a certain degree of adrenal suppression due to the continued high level of exogenous steroids. For patients who are no longer on steroids but who have had steroids in the past on any continuous basis, the question of possible adrenal suppression (even partial suppression) needs to be raised and evaluated. In any patient with adrenal suppression stress of any variety (i.e., surgery, trauma, infection) may precipitate adrenal crisis characterized by cardiovascular and respiratory collapse because of the adrenally suppressed patient's inability to mobilize endogenous steroids needed at times of stress. To avoid this potentially life-threatening problem, adrenally suppressed patients should receive increased levels of corticosteroids prior to, at the time of, and following surgical procedures. A patient's physician should be consulted prior to dental and surgical procedures regarding need for manipulation of steroid dosages. In truly adrenally suppressed patients (which can be determined by an ACTH adrenal stimulation test) hospitalization should be considered prior to surgical procedures.

Patients with hypercorticism or patients receiving high doses of steroids for various disease states have an increased susceptibility to infection and bleeding. Such patients may have easy bruisability from capillary fragility and may have a prolonged bleeding time. Patients on prolonged steroids, in addition to showing many of the features of Cushing's syndrome, have an increased susceptibility to peptic ulcer disease and may therefore be anemic from chronic gastrointestinal blood loss. Therefore, before surgical procedures, a complete blood count, platelet count and bleeding time should be performed. To avoid bleeding problems, good surgical technique and proper attention to hemostasis are required. If extensive surgical procedures are anticipated or if one is operating in an infected surgical field, antibiotic coverage may be advisable.

d. Pregnancy

The dentist will frequently be called upon to treat pregnant patients. Treatment of the pregnant patient should begin with consultation with the patient's obstetrician. Most dental procedures can be performed but they should be limited during the first trimester. Drugs and radiographs should be limited and used only when absolutely necessary, especially in the first trimester, because of their potential teratogenicity. The fetus should be shielded whenever any radiographs are taken. Local anesthetics are generally safe in the pregnant woman; however, when use of other drugs is anticipated clearance from the patient's obstetrician is necessary because of their possible teratogenic effects. Tetracycline should not be used in the pregnant woman because of its potential to stain the fetus' dentition.

VIII. Immunologic Diseases, Immunosuppression, Malignancy

Immunodeficiency disorders may be classified as primary or secondary. Primary immunodeficiency disorders are hereditary and include abnormalities of the B-cell line (abnormalities in humoral antibody production) and T-cell deficiency (abnormality in cellular immunity). Patients with B-cell deficiency are predisposed to frequent and recurrent bacterial infections, especially of the respiratory tract, and may see the dentist for recurrent sinusitis. Patients with T-cell deficiency are susceptible to frequent and recurrent viral and fungal infections and may present with oral candidiasis.

Secondary immune deficiency states can cause defects in the T-cell and B-cell lines of immunity. These states may be caused by granulomatous disease (i.e., tuberculosis or sarcoid), malignancy (especially leukemia, Hodgkin's disease, lymphoma and multiple myeloma, etc.), and chemotherapeutic agents used in the treatment of a variety of malignancies.

Management of immunosuppressed patients is difficult and requires a dentist-physician team approach. The main goal is to prevent and treat infection vigorously with close attention to culturing all infections for bacteria and fungi, followed by appropriate antibiotic therapy. Accurate culture techniques are important since these patients are susceptible to infection by unusual organisms; to provide specific antibiotic therapy one must identify the causative organism. Patients with B-cell deficiency may be getting immunoglobulins which may need to be increased prior to dental surgery or with significant dental infections. When treating immunosuppressed patients the dentist must familiarize himself with the patient's underlying disorder and the type of immune deficiency the patient may have. He must know what drugs the patient is taking and what effect they have on the immune system. This requires close contact with the patient's physician and these patients are generally best treated in a hospital setting where a multiple disciplinary approach is readily available.

Many causes of secondary immunodeficiency states (i.e., malignancy and drugs) affect not only the immune system but also the hematopoietic system. Many patients may therefore be anemic or thrombocytopenic and close attention must be paid to hemorrhage. Prior to surgical procedures, a complete blood count, platelet count and bleeding time should be ordered to determine the possibility of hemorrhage or presence of anemia. Various drugs may also affect liver function potentially causing prolonged prothrombin and partial thromboplastin time and an increased tendency for bleeding. When patients are taking such drugs clotting function studies should be measured prior to therapy.

The dentist can play a major role in the overall health of such patients since the oral cavity may be a potential source of infection in the immunosuppressed patient. Further studies are needed to confirm the oral cavity as a course of systemic infection in these patients. Ideally, if it is anticipated that a patient will require immunosuppressive agents, a complete oral examination and treatment of all sources of infection should be completed with the institution of preventive measures before immunosuppressive therapy is started. Periodic examination for signs of infection or drug toxicity should be performed on a regularly scheduled basis. This is also important for patients in whom radiation therapy to the head and neck is anticipated to prevent osteoradionecrosis of the jaw due to radiation-induced cellular and vascular damage to bone. As a result, all trauma and infection must be avoided in irradiated areas to prevent the development of osteoradionecrosis which may occur even years after radiation exposure. Patients who have had radiation to the head and neck should receive dental care from a practitioner experienced in this area.

IX. Autoimmune Disorders

The autoimmune disorders or collagen vascular disorders comprise a host of diseases that includes systemic lupus erythematosis, rheumatoid arthritis and many others. The diagnosis of many of these disorders is based on clinical findings–although various laboratory tests, for example, ESR, rheumatoid factor, antinuclear antibodies (ANA), are useful. Because these disorders are considered autoimmune, many of these patients are taking anti-inflammatory agents ranging from aspirin to steroids or immunosuppressive agents. When patients give a history of one of these disorders one must learn the extent of the patient's disease, what medication the patient is taking and take appropriate precautions. Medical consultation and evaluation prior to dental treatment are necessary in these patients. Patients with an exacerbation of one of these disorders or if extensive disease exists should be treated in a hospital setting.

a. Systemic Lupus Erythematosus (SLE)

SLE usually affects young females and is characterized by multiple organ involvement. Characteristic symptoms include various central nervous system symptoms, arthritis, renal insufficiency, anemia, pleuritis, and pericarditis, as well as many other symptoms. The differential diagnosis of any patient with oral ulcers must include SLE, especially when evidence of other organ involvement is present. Helpful laboratory tests in the diagnosis of SLE are the ANA, the ESR and the LE prep. When presented with a patient with a history of SLE, prior to dental treatment one must determine the extent of systemic organ involvement. Medical consultation is important. Many patients with SLE are taking aspirin or anti-inflammatory agents. Thus, bleeding problems secondary to abnormal platelet function or gastritis may occur. SLE itself may cause thrombocytopenia. Some patients have circulating anticoagulants and thus may have abnormal clotting studies. Prior to surgery a CBC, platelet count, prothrombin, partial thromboplastin and bleeding time should be performed. Many of these patients are taking steroids or immunosuppressant agents and may require their steroids to be increased prior to stressful procedures. If a patient is taking immunosuppressant agents, the preceding discussion regarding precautions to be taken with immunosuppressed patients needs to be considered. Surgical procedures and various drugs have been known to exacerbate SLE and, thus, only necessary drugs should be used and unnecessary surgery avoided.

b. Rheumatoid Arthritis (RA)

RA is a symmetrical polyarthritis characterized by pain, swelling, erythema and morning stiffness. Commonly affected joints are the MCP (metacarpal) and PIP (proximal interphalangeal) joints of the hands, wrists, elbows, knees and ankles. Extraarticular manifestations include subcutaneous nodules over extensor surfaces of the extremities, lymphadenopathy, splenomegaly, and less commonly, vasculitis, pleuritis, and pulmonary fibrosis and nodules. Laboratory findings include a positive rheumatoid factor and increased ESR. Variants of RA include Felty's syndrome, Still's disease, Sjögren's syndrome (characterized by lacrimal and salivary gland infiltration resulting in dry eyes and mouth) and Reiter's syndrome. Of dental concern is that RA may affect the temporomandibular joint, causing crepitus, stiffness, pain and even ankylosis. Medical consultation is needed in these patients. They may also be taking a variety of anti-inflammatory and immunosuppressant agents so appropriate precautions must be taken. Some patients will be taking gold salts which may result in stomatitis and oral ulcers.

Other less common autoimmune diseases include polymyalgia rheumatica, polymyositis, scleroderma, and thyroiditis, as well as many others. When a patient gives a history of any of these disorders, medical consultation is necessary to determine the extent of the patient's disease, the medications he is taking, and what precautions are necessary prior to dental treatment.

X. Hematologic Abnormalities

The main concerns a dentist will have when treating patients with hematologic disorders are patients with anemia and bleeding problems which may be secondary to any number of underlying causes.

a. Anemia

One should suspect the diagnosis of anemia in any patient who has pallor of the skin, mucous membranes or nail beds or who complains of fatigue or weakness. The diagnosis may be confirmed by determining the patient's hematocrit which can be done in the dentist's office. There are multiple forms of anemia with many different causes and therapies. Various malignancies (hematologic or otherwise) and chronic diseases can cause anemia. These have already been discussed in the section on immunosuppression. Patients with chronic blood loss, iron deficiency or vitamin deficiency may be anemic. Various drugs and autoimmune disorders may cause a hemolytic anemia.

In any patient with a history or suspicion of anemia, various diagnostic tests are indicated, beginning with evaluation of the blood smear and complete blood count. If a patient is found to be anemic, medical consultation is required for further diagnostic evaluation regarding the type of anemia, its cause and treatment, and how it may affect or be affected by dental procedures.

b. Bleeding Disorders

There are many causes of bleeding problems. They may be due to clotting factor abnormalities, abnormal platelet number or function, or capillary fragility. All dental patients should be questioned regarding a history of bleeding abnormalities. Patients should be questioned regarding bleeding following surgery or tooth extractions, spontaneous bleeding from nose, gingiva (more than can be accounted for by local factors), genitourinary tract, purpura or petechia. Patients who give a history of or symptoms or signs of a bleeding problem need (prior to dental treatment) medical referral for further evaluation consisting of a complete blood count, platelet count, prothrombin, partial thromboplastin and bleeding times to determine the underlying cause for the bleeding abnormality and its treatment. The specific dental management of patients with underlying bleeding problems is discussed in the chapter dealing with office emergencies. As discussed in this chapter, there are some patients who will be taking anticoagulants, usually Coumadin, for various medical reasons. A patient's physician should always be consulted when the patient is taking these drugs. These drugs are vitamin K antagonists and inhibit production by the liver of clotting factors II, VII, IX and X. The degree of anticoagulation can be measured by the prothrombin time which is usually kept 1½ to 2 times control. Many oral surgeons feel a prothrombin time 1½ times control is acceptable for minor surgical procedures. If major surgical procedures are anticipated, anticoagulants should be stopped 72 hours prior to surgery. This should be done only with physician consultation because patients who absolutely need anticoagulation may have to be hospitalized and switched to heparin, which is rapid-acting, with a short half life, and can be stopped or reversed with protamine just before surgery and reinstituted after surgery. Later, Coumadin can be restarted. The effect of Coumadin can be reversed with vitamin K which takes 12 to 24 hours. In emergency situations, patients can be given fresh frozen plasma or factor concentrate to replace the factors affected by Coumadin.

chapter

4

Office Emergencies and Statim Medical Complications

LEVENTE Z. BODAK-GYOVAI

I. Useful Medications and Equipment

The best "treatment" of a medical problem or emergency complication in a dental office is prevention: obtaining and routinely updating the detailed anamnesis, vital signs, familiarity with all the essential, pertinent diagnoses and medications, preparing careful dental treatment plans in cooperation with the patient's physician, if necessary, in compromised medical cases, considering drug contraindications, side effects and interactions. This preventive thinking is the only proper patient management concept to avoid, whenever possible, the need for medical emergency treatment.

Keep all the established modern and new emergency aids at hand when engaging in dental treatment.

1. Medication: since extreme anxiety, fear and stress can elicit complications and emergencies in the patients with compromised medical status, it is wise to allay their emotional reactions by using the technique of premedication:

Valium (diazepam), 2, 5, 10 mg tablets.

Nembutal sodium (pentobarbital-sodium), 30, 50 mg capsules.

Seconal sodium (secobarbital-sodium), 30, 50 mg capsules.

Phenergan (promethazine hydrochloride), 12.5, 25, 50 mg tablets (sedative, antihistaminic and antiemetic action).

Demerol hydrochloride (meperidine hydrochloride), 50, 100 mg tablets 2.5% (25 mg per ml) Carpuject for parenteral use (narcotic analgesic, sedative).

Benadryl (diphenhydramine hydrochloride), 25 mg capsules, 50 mg per 1 ml Parke-Davis premade disposable syringe; 22 gauge, 1-inch needle (sedative, antiemetic, antihistamine, antispasmodic/anticholinergic).

Dilantin (phenytoin sodium), 30, 100 mg capsules, 50 mg per ml in a 2 ml sterile disposable (Parke-Davis) syringe; 22 gauge, 1¼-inch needle (anticonvulsant).

Narcotic reversal: Narcan (naloxone hydrochloride) 0.4 mg per 1 ml ampules, IV, IM, SC.

Amyl nitrite inhalant, 0.18, 0.3 ml Aspirol buds (relief of angina pectoris).

Nitrostat (nitroglycerin), 0.15, 0.3, 0.4, 0.6 mg sublingual tablets (angina pectoris).

Xylocaine (lidocaine hydrochloride), intramuscular injection for cardiac arrhythmias, 100 mg per ml in 5 ml ampules.

Isuprel hydrochloride (isoproterenol hydrochloride), 0.2 mg per 1 ml ampules and 1 mg per 5 ml ampules (bronchodilator, relaxes GI tract, increases cardiac output, venous return, i.e., elevating systolic BP, vasopressor, therefore, used in bronchospasm, cardiac arrest, arrhythmia, shock).

Isuprel hydrochloride Mistometer, 15 ml nebulizing unit (bronchodilator), or

Medihaler-Iso (isoproterenol sulfate) 15 ml aerosol spray (bronchodilator).

Aminophyllin (aminophylline) 100 mg tablets, 500 mg per 2 ml ampules, IM, or 250 mg per 10 ml ampules, IV, 22 gauge, 1-inch needle (bronchodilator).

Adrenalin chloride (epinephrine), 1 mg per 1 ml ampules, IM, IV, SC, intracardially for cardiac resuscitation (1:1000 prepared Parke-Davis "TB" syringe) (vasopressor/sympathomimetic) or epinephrine 1:10,000 per 10 ml Abboject injection.

Neo-Synephrine hydrochloride (phenylephrine hydrochloride), 10 mg per 1 ml ampules (1%) (vasoconstrictor).

Atropine sulfate, 0.4 mg per 1 ml (20 ml ampules), 22 gauge, 1-inch needle, IM, 0.4 mg tablets (anticholinergic).

Solu-Cortef (hydrocortisone sodium succinate), 100 mg plain vials, 100 mg Mix-O-Vial, 2-ml syringe, 22 gauge, 1-inch needle, IV, IM.

Decadron phosphate (dexamethasone sodium phosphate), 4 mg per 1 ml disposable syringes, prepared by Merck Sharp & Dohme, IV, IM, intraarticular, SC.

0.9% (N) Saline solution, 1000 ml bottles, bags, IV infusion.

Dextran 70 injection, 6% dextran 70 in 0.9% sodium chloride, 250 and 500 ml (plasma volume expander).

Dextran 40 injection, 10% dextran 40 in 5% dextrose, 500 ml (or in 0.9% sodium chloride, 500 ml) for IV infusion.

50% Dextrose, 50 ml ampules, 18 gauge, 1-inch needle, IV.

Calcium Disodium Versenate (calcium disodium edetate), 200 mg per 1 ml (20%) in 5 ml ampules, IV, IM.

Sodium bicarbonate, 7.5%, 50 ml (44.6 mEq per liter solution), 22 gauge, 1-inch needle.

Lactated ringer with 5% dextrose, IV infusion (D5LR, 250 ml).

Spirits of ammonia (ammonia inhalant pearls).

2. The following equipment and instruments must be readily available in excellent working order.

Stethoscope with sphygmomanometer and BP cuff.

Positive pressure oxygen device with adapters.

Plastic oropharyngeal airways of all sizes (disposable airway no. 2, 3 and 4).

Nasopharyngeal tubes.

Curved cricothyrotomy cannula.

Respiratory pressure reservoir bag, Ambu-bag, paper bag, and Laerdal packet mask in child and adult sizes.

Tourniquet.

No. 3, 21 gauge Butterfly Infusion set with tubing and cannula for IV drug administration (Longdwell No. 880-35, Teflon over the needle).

Syringes 1, 10, 20, 50 ml.

Vacutainer tubes with adjuvants.

H.V.E. (proper suction).

Oxygen (tank, regulator, flowmeter).

Towel clips and ice bag.

Paper tape, ½-inch roll.

Mouth prop (rubber protected).

Ring forceps, padded tongue blade, metal tongue depressor.

2 inch x 2 inch alcohol gauze.

3. Telephone numbers.

Nearest hospital emergency ward.

Nearest ambulance service, police or fire department.

Patient's physician.

Nearest medical practitioner.

Medicolegally, the dentist is not obliged to engage in the treatment and management of patients' medical complications or emergencies, but the dentist must provide emergency first aid in the dental office as well as outside of the office.

It is of utmost importance to realize that there is a medical complication or emergency situation present. This emergency problem can be aggravated if the dentist is not well versed in proper patient management. For example, if the patient goes into unconsciousness following local anesthesia, N_2O analgesia and develops respiratory failure, no time should be wasted in determining whether the reaction was allergic, toxic or disease related (i.e., the patient has a history of bronchial asthma and recent upper respiratory tract infection). In such cases, the delivery of indicated emergency patient management is essential. In general, most emergency life-threatening situations are induced by abnormal reactions to drugs, interactions between various medications, emotional (or physical) stress or compromised medical status (i.e., complications related to preexisting systemic disorders, such as cardiopulmonary diseases).

When the patient is unable to withstand, cope with and successfully overcome the effects of various deleterious hazards, the emergency life-supporting measures may help the patient's survival. Place the patient, if possible, in a supine position and insure the following:

A. Unobliterated *airway* (eliminate the blocking artifact, if necessary).

B. Efficient *breathing* (maintain artificial respiration, if indicated).

C. Adequate blood *circulation* by detecting the central (carotid) pulse, and restore blood circulation by administering cardiopulmonary resuscitation (CPR) if the central pulse is absent.

II. Description of Signs, Symptoms and Management of the Medical Complications in the Dental Office

To facilitate the use of this book alphabetical order is followed.

Acute Adrenal Crisis

Acute adrenal crisis is a rapid and overwhelming exacerbation of chronic adrenal insufficiency. Chronic adrenal insufficiency is characterized by the following signs and symptoms: insidious onset, weakness, progressive fatigability, nausea, vomiting, anorexia, weight loss, cutaneous and mucosal pigmentation, hypotension and sometimes hypoglycemia.

In the untreated patient the preexisting symptoms are intensified: nausea, vomiting and abdominal pain (may become intractable), fever (frequently severe), lethargy (quickly deepens), the blood pressure and pulse fall, and hypovolemic shock ensues. The concurrence of infection, trauma (including surgery), gastrointestinal upset or other forms of stress demands an immediate increase in output of adrenal hormones, and the survival of patients with Addison's disease may depend upon treat-

ment of an acute crisis. Prevention of the crisis consists of adequate steroid supplements, if necessary.

The treatment is mainly directed toward the elevation of circulating adrenocortical hormones, in addition to the replacement of the sodium and water deficit. An IV infusion of 1,000 ml, 5% glucose in normal saline solution containing 100 to 200 mg of any of the several soluble hydrocortisone preparations is recommended. If the crisis was preceded by prolonged nausea and vomiting much of the normal saline replacement is indicated.

Acute Barbiturate Intoxication

Acute barbiturate poisoning is an overdose of the derivatives of barbituric acid. Moderately severe poisoning occurs with ingestion of 5 to 10 times the full hypnotic dose, and death is liable to occur with 15 to 20 times of this amount. Administration of CNS depressants gravely aggravates the situation.

Signs and symptoms of moderate intoxication are as follows. The patient may move on painful stimulation, respiration is slow, gag reflex is depressed, the pupils may be slightly constricted and usually react to light; rarely they may be markedly constricted (miosis) as in morphine poisoning; deep tendon reflexes are preserved, drowsiness, mental confusion, hallucinations, and slurred speech are present, the pulse is weak. In severe intoxication, no response to pain or vigorous manual stimulation is seen, pupils may be dilated (mydriasis) and may not react to light. Both gag and cough reflexes are absent, deep tendon reflexes are usually absent but sometimes are hyperactive, respiration is slow and shallow, cyanosis is obvious, the temperature and the blood pressure are low.

The therapy should be directed to maintaining an open airway, providing adequate respiration and circulation, along with combating shock. Immediate measures are: remove dentures, if present, insert oral airway, place the patient on his side with his head downward. Give mouth-to-mouth (and CPR), if necessary. Transport the patient to the hospital emergency ward.

Acute Bronchial (Pulmonary) Asthmatic Attack

Asthma is characterized by expiratory wheezing, expiratory dyspnea (prolonged expiratory phase), severe chest pain, early nonproductive cough and late thick mucous sputum production; in severe cases there is a sense of suffocation, overinflation of the lungs, distended chest and cyanosis. Bronchial and bronchiolar airway obstruction occurs as a result of contraction of bronchial smooth muscles, hypertrophy of the bronchial mucosa, and accumulation of mucous secretion in the lumen of bronchi throughout the bronchopulmonary segments.

In the development of asthmatic attacks there is a certain degree of interaction of the following factors:

Polluted air.

Hypersensitivity to inhaled allergens.

Infection of the respiratory tract.

Stress related psychological response.

Constitutional predisposition to allergic reactions.

Dyspnea is most pronounced and wheezing is most audible by auscultation during prolonged expiration and cough throughout the chest; these manifestations are worse with effort, exaggerated by anxiety and stress, and tend to be most severe at night. Syncope may occur during prolonged periods of the attack. Asthma occurs in attacks; between attacks the patient is free of symptoms. Spasmodic asthma is more frequent at night, and attacks usually last several minutes to hours. After a prolonged attack the patient will complain of soreness in the chest or abdomen as well as profound tiredness. During an attack, the patient is most comfortable while sitting with the trunk forward and the arms elevated to rest at shoulder level.

The ease with which sputum can be evacuated from the bronchi is an important factor in the severity of airway obstruction. The physical properties of the bronchial secretions are influencing the manifestations of the attack of asthma. When the sputum seems to be more liquid, and is present in larger quantities the cough becomes more severe during the recovery from an asthmatic attack. The sputum is usually white, mucoid and may contain eosinophils. Purulent sputum indicates bronchial infection. There is no fever unless asthma is associated with infection. Moist pulmonary rales, blood-tinged sputum and cardiac decompensation may be related to pulmonary edema causing cardiac asthma.

During a mild attack the sensation of airway obstruction may lead the patient to overcompensate by hyperpnea. If airway obstruction becomes more severe, there is a fall in oxygen tension of blood with cyanosis and a rise in CO_2 partial pressure in developing the ventilatory (respiratory) failure.

When an asthmatic episode is prolonged (hours) and is resistant to therapy, it is defined as status asthmaticus. The chest is distended and wheezes become very faint because movement of air is poor (diminished ventilation). Cough is impossible and the patient is extremely fatigued, prostrate. If the status doesn't improve, the chest becomes almost silent, severe respiratory acidosis sets in and death from respiratory arrest is possible.

Emergency therapy: the mild attacks are readily relieved by inhalation of nebulized isoproterenol, Isuprel Mistometer (1 to 2 deep inhalations) while the patient is in an upright, sitting position. The smallest effective amount should be used, if possible every three hours. In case of a rapidly developing attack, 0.3 to 0.5 ml of 1:1,000 epinephrine should be injected SC; the dose may be repeated every 30 minutes, p.r.n. In case of severe dyspnea and cyanosis, give oxygen support. Older patients should receive 0.25 mg of terbutaline SC since it has less effect on the cardiovascular system than epinephrine.

At the time of onset of asthmatic attacks, a sedative, e.g., amobarbital (50 to 100 mg) can be used to cope with agitation and anxiety. In order to avoid respiratory failure and sudden death, the respiratory depressants, e.g., morphine, should not be used during asthmatic episodes.

Aminophylline (theophylline ethylenediamine) may be used (dose of 0.25 gm, IV, or rectally, administered over a 20-minute period) for adequate bronchodilation. If the patient has been taking aminophylline on a regular basis a smaller dose (0.9 mg/kg per hr) should be used.

In relieving bronchospasm the administration of corticosteroids may be necessary, e.g., prednisone 15 to 80 mg per day, or hydrocortisone sodium succinate (Solu-Cortef), 100 to 300 mg IV. The steroids should be continued to maintain improvement and then tapered. Preventive administration of steroids to patients with chronic asthma or asthmatic bronchitis is considered to be effective in controlling the attacks. Similar considerations may indicate the use of aminophylline, 200 mg, P.O., t.i.d., or terbutaline, 5 mg, P.O., t.i.d. or q.i.d., prior to dental surgery.

If cholinergic drug poisoning related dyspnea is recognized atropine should relieve the bronchoconstriction.

Acute Fulminant Infections Involving Heart Valves

Acute fulminant infections involving heart valves is a condition of overwhelming pyogenic bacterial infection invading the heart valves or damaged endocardial surface of congenital abnormalities of the heart. The microbes are not destroyed, since there is a lack of bodily defense to invasion of bacteria when this condition occurs.

The symptoms depend on the nature of the organisms and the underlying cardiac lesion: petechiae, emboli, pyrexia, anemia, cardiac symptoms, cerebral vascular lesion, subacute rheumatism, nephritis and bronchopneumonia are common. The spleen is usually palpable. The history of dental sepsis (recent tooth extraction, other surgical procedures in the oral region) is elicited in 48% of all cases. The untreated patient may die within a few days due to septicemia or embolism.

The therapy includes specific antibiotics, e.g., penicillin and streptomycin in large parenteral doses daily for 6 to 8 weeks. This preferred treatment may be effective in 90% of cases.

Acute Hemorrhage

Both hemorrhage and control following surgical procedures are undoubtedly one of the most common and serious complications encountered by the dental practitioner.

Injury and trauma to blood vessels may result in acute extravasation of blood, and the bleeding complications may be the results of the following defects:

1. Unavailability of any of the precursor substances involved in coagulation.
2. Absence of any of the coagulation factors.
3. Interference with any phases of normal hemostatic, coagulation and lysis systems.
4. Drug interaction with clotting mechanisms.

The essential preoperative prophylactic measures of hemorrhagic problems include a complete patient's history, examination and laboratory tests when a bleeding abnormality is suspected. The patient's history should extend to questions regarding previous bleeding experiences, results of former tooth extractions and surgeries, i.e., whether there is a history of spontaneous, easy purpura, epistaxis, excessive bleeding for a relatively prolonged time from minor cuts or wounds. The history of any of the hemorrhagic disorders, blood dyscrasias, leukemia or familial bleeding tendencies (hemophilia) should be thoroughly evaluated. The menstrual history is significant since the postoperative bleeding may emerge if the patient has menorrhagia (prolonged and profuse menstrual hemorrhage), or metrorrhagia (abnormal uterine bleeding). Preventive measures should include preoperative radiographs in the area of surgery, since these may indicate closely related normal or aberrant blood vessels or abnormally dilated nutrient arteries.

Medications taken by the patient are also important concerning the hemorrhage, e.g., hormones, iron preparations for anemia, salicylates, and anticoagulants.

Peptic ulcer is one of the most common causes of acute internal hemorrhage: bleeding into the gastrointestinal tract may be the cause of unexplained weakness, faintness, unconsciousness, syncope with or without pain, hematemesis or melena.

The physical examination should describe the appearance of the skin and the color of the eyes (jaundice), nail beds, lips, gingivae, the presence of petechiae, tenderness of bones and joints, in order to dispose a bleeding tendency, anemia, liver disease, leukemia, etc. There are several types of hemorrhages based on the appearance of the bleeding:

1. Capillary = steady oozing, bright red.
2. Vascular bed, e.g., hemangioma = profuse, darker red.
3. Arterial = intermittent pumping, bright red.
4. Venous = steady flow, bluish red.

Local control of hemorrhage is intended to arrest bleeding long enough to form a clot, a "mechanical plug" to occlude the lumen of vessels. Topical agents such as epinephrine can be effective, applied in 1:1,000 concentrations, carried on a piece of gauze, or injected locally in 1:50,000 concentration, but care should be exercised in case of existing cardiovascular disease, ischemic heart disease, angina pectoris, myocardial infarct, severe hypertension. Other topical hemostatic and vasoconstrictor agents include Surgicel, Gelfoam, Monsel's solution (ferric subsulfate), tea bag (tannic acid) or ice application. Suturing the wound over oxidized cellulose or absorbable gelatin sponge moistened with thrombin solution can also effectively reduce hemorrhage.

Following an extraction, and removal of the raw exposed edges of bone and bone fragments and inserting the suture(s), a rolled pack of dry sponge (gauze) is placed directly over the alveolar area, permitting the patient to bite firmly. This method should control the hemorrhage in 10 to 15 minutes. Sometimes it is necessary to dress the alveolar socket tightly with a gauze or sponge to apply pressure counteracting the hydrostatic pressure within the bleeding vessels until a clot can form, obturate the vessel lumen and stop the hemorrhage. Bone wax and bone punch are other mechanical measures to cope with bleeding from bone. The postextraction alveolar hemorrhage of a simple single tooth removal can be easily controlled by having the patient bite firmly on a pad of folded gauze for a period of 15 minutes.

Hemorrhage from soft tissue wounds, cuts or incisions may be controlled by applying pressure directly over the injured area, or indirectly on a pressure point of the regional artery till clot can form (5 to 10 minutes without removing the pressure or dressing to see if the bleeding has stopped!). In case of surgical procedures the avoidance of soft tissue tearing, careful dissection, clamping and ligating any of the bleeding blood vessels and placing the sutures properly (without tension) are essential steps in the control of hemorrhage. If the patient is accidentally wounded and the patient's general condition permits, it is important to determine the exact site which bleeding is occurring by removing the coagulated blood (suction), washing the wound with warm, sterile, saline solution and brushing out (following a good local anesthesia) all of the foreign materials. The patient's general condition should be monitored and the adequacy of the circulation (blood pressure and pulse) should be determined. If signs of shock are seen (low blood pressure, rapid, weak pulse, cold, clammy, pale skin, cyanotic ears, lips, mucous membranes, etc.) autotransfusion (place the patient's head lower than the feet) should be instituted, followed by intravenous fluids and blood. Be sure that the airways are not obstructed by clots of blood.

Considering good postoperative care for oral surgical procedures the following can be included: in patients with preexisting blood dyscrasias, hemophilia, or mental retardation (the patient may remove the clot, suture) a splint is to be worn by the patient, or wired in place over the surgical area and adequate postoperative sedation should be provided at a level to maintain cough reflex. In order not to allow blood to seep into the trachea elevate the head by placing the patient in a secured sitting position.

For systemic control of hemorrhage, agents such as transfusion of whole blood, fresh frozen plasma, vitamin K and fibrinogen are commonly employed. To arrest epistaxis press the nostril or the bleeding site for a few minutes, apply cold to the nose, ask the patient to breathe through the mouth, then plug the nose with lubricated gauze, leaving the gauze to hang out of the nostril, and instruct the patient not to blow the nose for hours.

Acute Hypertensive Crisis

Arterial hypertension is a disease condition characterized by persistent elevation in recorded blood pressure. In this disease entity the systolic or diastolic pressure or both are elevated. The potential role of the dental profession is unique in that it is possible to provide adequate medical evaluation in suspected hypertensive cases, to express a cooperative effort in controlling hypertension by physicians, and help to reduce the illnesses and mortality (1.5 million per year in the U.S.A.) attributable to high blood pressure. In providing quality dental care the high blood pressure state requires careful treatment planning, including consideration of premedication (stress), selection of an anesthetic (vasoconstrictor) and determining the extent and duration of operative procedures. It has been estimated that 20% of the entire U.S. population and one out of every four patients over 40 years of age who enter a dental office has some form of high arterial blood pressure, a disease which is primarily asymptomic, but may result in the early phase of cardiac complications, cerebrovascular accident, renal disease or retinal hemorrhage as the clear outcome of undetected, therefore, uncontrolled severe hypertension. The increasingly aging population (resulting from factors such as advancing medical sciences, patient care, etc.) increases the number of both hypertensive and dental patients. More and more patients are treated successfully for angina pectoris, myocardial infarction, congestive heart failure, etc., and they come to the dental office to obtain elective (or emergency) services. Hypertensive patients, focusing attention on the disease, are usually more easily upset emotionally, developing greater than acceptable levels of morbidity during the anticipated dental procedure that may be a real threat. These patients can overreact to pressure stimulation with distinctly high changes in blood pressure. A patient with hypertension may account for an occasional sudden death in the dental office, therefore, it is essential to identify the person with severe uncontrolled hypertension prior to dental surgery/operative procedures, since apprehension, stress, anxiety and nervous tension can precipitate a critical rise in blood pressure, the acute hypertensive crisis. Patients with hypertensive disease may suffer from acute "spontaneous" episodes of marked, sudden elevation in blood pressure associated with disorders of the central nervous system. The state of acute hypertensive crisis, hypertensive encephalopathy can last from minutes to days, and may disappear without clinical evidences of lasting damage.

The generalized form of acute hypertensive crisis, aside from the rapidly rising blood pressure, is characterized by severe headache, visual disturbances (papilloedema), vomiting, congestive heart failure, psychoses, convulsions, stupor and coma.

The focal form of acute hypertensive crisis is characterized by focal disturbances in the central nervous system, with various clinical manifestations such as loss of consciousness, convulsions and paralysis involving one half of the body. Although reversible, it may exactly resemble the clinical picture of cerebrovascular accident caused by hemorrhage, embolism or thrombosis. Differential diagnosis is possible if several hours elapse with the patient under careful observation. The focal form is most frequent in elderly individuals having either chronic or malignant hypertensive vascular disease.

In either form of the hypertensive condition, the onset of clinical manifestations is initiated and hastened by apprehension, worry, anxiety, pain and fear, excessive fluid input, long, fatiguing appointments, multiple stressful extractions, extensive dental surgical procedures and protracted dental manipulations of "mild" nature. Therefore, management of the patient should begin with preventive measures to prevent anxiety by employing premedication (tranquilizers, sedatives) and a good local anesthesia (aspirating cartridge syringes, a low level of vasoconstrictor content in the local anesthetic solution, fine gauge of needles, prior topical anesthetic, etc.), and utilizing the psychosomatic effects of "vocal anesthesia" keeping a close and excellent level of rapport with the patient. Avoid the use of general anesthetic agents; this is related to an extremely high and certain degree of risk involved in patients with arterial hypertension to develop the condition of acute hypertensive crisis or hypertensive encephalopathy, which may be resistant to correction during general anesthesia. Drug interaction related to antihypertensive medications is always a realistic possibility mandating adjustment of doses of various drugs used in general dental practice (see Appendix II).

During a hypertensive crisis of left ventricular failure with acute pulmonary edema, the following clinical signs and symptoms are predominant: dyspnea, cough with frothy sputum, hemoptysis, vertigo and precordial pain. Management of the patient with acute hypertensive crisis (or acute pulmonary edema) is a medical emergency and consists of quick lowering of the blood pressure by pharmacologic means, including:

Furosemide, 40 to 400 mg IV (diuresis).

Diazoxide, 300 mg IV (diabetogenic).

Sodium nitroprusside.

Management of hypertensive crisis requires an emergency medical facility where close medical management and monitoring can be performed.

Acute Respiratory Failure and Arrest

When respiratory failure is present the partial pressure of carbon dioxide is elevated (above 35 to 45 mm Hg) and the oxygen is decreased (below 80 to 100 mm Hg) in the arterial blood. This can commence with the malfunctions of the following systems: respiratory system (external respiration, the absorption of oxygen from the atmosphere and elimination of carbon dioxide from the pulmonary alveolar vessels); circulatory system (internal respiration, the exchange of oxygen and carbon dioxide takes place between the capillary blood and tissues in the environment of these small blood vessels).

Many of the central nervous system disorders, as well as the direct destruction, damage or functional depression of neurons in the respiratory center can produce rapidly developing central respiratory failure or arrest. Certain diseases, e.g., poliomyelitis, encephalitis or drugs, e.g., opiates, CNS depressants (barbiturates, Valium, Librium) are frequent causes of central respiratory failure.

Disorders of the peripheral nervous system, damage to the motor tracts and branches from the spinal cord, nerve pathways to the respiratory muscles and the respiratory muscles themselves, or anatomic structures associated with respira-

tion (i.e., airway obstruction, or pneumothorax) can result in peripheral respiratory failure. (Suffocation, asphyxia and drowning are some extreme cases of acute respiratory "failure"/respiratory arrest).

In acute respiratory failure the following is seen: dyspnea, slow, irregular and superficial respiration, or gasping. Acute respiratory failure can lead to respiratory arrest which in turn results in cardiac arrest.

If airway obstruction is present the conscious patient gags, coughs, exhibits "noisy labored" breathing, strains the neck, chest and abdominal muscles, chokes, and rapidly develops cyanosis of the skin and mucous membranes.

If an upper respiratory tract obstruction is present and the patient is conscious, lower the head, turn the patient lateral in the chair, bring the mandible in a protruded-open position. If the patient is unconscious use—in addition—a mechanical airway. This position may hamper slightly the respiration of an obese patient. If the obstructing foreign body cannot be removed from the upper respiratory tract region by instruments (forceps, suction) or the Heimlich maneuver (sudden, forceful pressure above the umbilical area) the lifesaving coniotomy (or tracheostomy) should be considered. Mouth-to-mouth (or airway) resuscitation or artificial equipment respiration (positive pressure oxygen) is to be used as follows if there is respiratory difficulty without obliteration of the upper respiratory tract:

Airway is opened by tilting the head back.

Breathing is assured, 12 to 16 times per minute.

In the case of drug induced, CNS depression related apnea:

Trendelenburg position.

Positive pressure oxygen or artificial respiration.

Analeptics to keep patient awake.

Consider Naloxone hydrochloride (Narcan), 0.4 mg IV, IM, SC if narcotic overdose is to be reversed.

Adequate blood circulation.

Monitor vital signs and transport patient to the hospital emergency ward.

Alcohol Intoxication

Alcoholism is the state of addiction to alcohol, the excessive consumption of alcohol. Neither cause nor cure is known for alcoholism. It is a syndrome in which physiologic, biochemical, psychologic and cultural factors play highly significant (though not clearly understood) roles.

The signs and symptoms of clinical abnormalities result from the physiologic effect of ethyl alcohol, e.g., a local irritant when taken into the stomach in any sizable quantities, acting as a strong depressant on the CNS. The early removal of inhibitions is followed by gradual impairment of judgment, the reflexes are markedly slowed and lack of coordination is characteristic. Further absorption of alcohol gradually exceeds the rate at which the body can metabolize it and a toxic condition is reached; at this point the depression of the CNS has become severe, the patient is pale, has cold sweats, probably vomits, shows signs of shock and lapses into unconsciousness. A fatal outcome is possible. Mild acute intoxication is characterized by euphoria, decreased inhibitions (mental, physical), urge of combative actions, decreased ability to perform coordinated, rapid, repetitive muscle acts, slight tremor, ataxia, increased reflex time, lessened sense of fatigue, slight visual impairment. Moderate acute intoxication is described as causing emotional lability, memory deficit, clumsiness, drowsiness, blurred vision and slurred speech, nausea, dyspnea, flushing, elevated pain threshold and definite ataxia. In heavy acute intoxication the muscle incoordination is prominent, the respiration is slow and deep, the pulse rate is elevated, pupils exhibit mydriasis, and diplopia is present; the reflexes are diminished, the response to painful stimulation is feeble, the skin is cold and clammy, and coma and death may commence due to respiratory arrest.

The treatment of a case of average mild inebriation should be supportive and the victim would need several hours of sleep to metabolize and eliminate the ingested alcohol.

The moderate and severe alcohol intoxication may require definite therapy: inducing vomiting to empty and wash out the stomach (gastric lavage or "stomach pumping") with normal saline solution (less than 1 teaspoon of table salt in more than a large glass of water), to evacuate the remaining alcohol from the stomach,

and to palliate the alcoholic gastritis. A large dose of Epsom salt or other saline cathartic solution should be administered to purge the intestinal tract. To prevent the development of shock and pneumonia the patient should be kept warm and given IV fluids.

Allergic Reaction and Toxic Overdose of Local Anesthetics

Drug allergy is a specific hypersensitivity reaction of the sensitized patient; the patient may exhibit mild to severe allergic reaction characterized by various degrees of urticaria, pruritus or angioneurotic edema (edematous swelling of hands, the periorbital areas, eyelids, lips, tongue, other extraoral and intraoral facial structures, pharynx and laryngeal edema). The clinical manifestations can progress to anaphylactic shock (profound hypotension, hoarseness, asphyxia sensation, mydriasis, cyanosis, loss of consciousness and wheezing dyspnea). To prevent an allergic reaction one should inquire about the patient's sensitivity to the drug or chemical agent prior to its administration. Usually the patient has an allergic history, secondary to exposure to allergens. Mild or severe allergic reactions may involve the skin, mucous membranes or blood vessels, resulting in skin exanthems, pruritus, urticaria, rhinitis, rhinorrhea, asthma (respiratory difficulties, expiratory dyspnea with short, gasping inspiration and prolonged expiration, bronchial smooth muscle spasm) or angioneurotic edema. The allergic response may be the immediate or delayed type. An anaphylactic shock (hypotension from vasodilation) is rare but constitutes an extreme emergency (see under Anaphylactic Shock).

Toxic overdose of a local anesthetic may occur as a result of administration of large doses of the local anesthetic (13 capsules of 1.8 ml per 2% sol. = 468 mg) in high concentration, increased rate of absorption and diffusion influenced by the technique (how fast the amount of drug is given), route of drug administration (possibility of an inadvertent intravascular injection), decreased drug metabolism, detoxification (biotransformation) and slow rate of elimination of end products. The patient's general medical condition, emotional status and other drugs administered may efficiently enhance the development of systemic toxic reactions to the local anesthetic.

An early manifestation is that of overstimulation of the central nervous system, including apprehension, disorientation, excitement, convulsions, altered vital signs. Stimulation of the central nervous system may be followed by depression (can be the primary outcome), decreased blood pressure, tachypnea, rapid weak pulse, lethargy, drowsiness, decrease of superficial and deep reflexes, visual disturbances, miosis, confusion, convulsions, onset of bradycardia, unconsciousness, stupor, coma, peripheral vascular collapse and depression of the respiratory center (apnea, cyanosis), which may lead to death.

The general routine prevention of complications should include aspiration during injection, slow drug administration, the lowest concentration of vasoconstrictor recommended, the smallest effective amount of local anesthetic solution used and premedication to avoid anxiety and agitation.

Therapy of an allergic response should correspond to the reaction experienced. If the allergic reaction is severe, involving the tracheobronchial tree, the treatment should include administration of oxygen, epinephrine-HCl (Adrenalin) in 1:1,000 concentration, 0.3 to 0.5 ml, SC, repeated in 5 to 10 minutes if needed (the epinephrine will improve cardiac tone, raise the blood pressure, relieve edema and pruritus and reduce bronchospasm).

Bronchospasm can be quickly relieved by Aminophylline (theophylline ethylenediamine), 250 m IV given very slowly; Solu-Cortef (hydrocortisone sodium succinate) 100 mg, or Decadron (dexamethasone sodium phosphate) 4 mg IV or IM. Oxygen should also be administered through an adequate airway; Trendelenburg position. If sustained convulsions occur anticonvulsants should be given IV.

In most cases the early reaction to toxic overdose of local anesthetics is immediate, mild and short-lasting with complete recovery without the requirement of treatment. In case the patient passes from the CNS excitation to depression, the administration of 100% oxygen is suggested (10 liter flow) to support respiration and prevent respiratory depression. Sympathomimetics can be given, e.g., Adrenalin (epinephrine-HCl) in 1 mg per 1 ml (1:1,000) concentration 0.2 to 0.5 ml SC, or Levophed (levarterenol bitartrate), 1 mg per 1 ml solution IV, with intravenous fluids, e.g., 5% dextrose in saline solution (add 4 ml of Levophed to 1,000 ml of 5% dextrose solution = 4 μg Levophed in 1 ml dilution) given through IV catheter. Give Atropine, 0.6 mg IV for severe bradycardia. Start CPR, if indicated, consider coniotomy, if necessary. Any type of allergic reaction noted needs to have written evidence in the patient's chart. The patient's vital signs should be monitored throughout the resuscitative measures. Medical help obviously must be sought.

Anaphylactic Shock

Anaphylaxis is a rapid, grave, immediate type of allergic reaction characteristically occurring upon administration (most often injection) of an antigen, e.g., foreign serum, medication such as penicillin (IM aqueous PCN is most frequently implicated) into the host with or without a history of previous exposure to the antigen induced hypersensitivity. The most likely candidates suffer from hay fever, asthma, drug, food or pollen allergies. This acute hypersensitivity reaction sometimes represents the cause of sudden death within minutes, due to the allergic involvement and impairment of the cardiovascular and respiratory (laryngo-tracheo-bronchopulmonary) systems. The typical clinical manifestations of anaphylactic shock may begin with the patient's complaints of a sense of uneasiness, apprehension; becoming agitated, flushed (to be differentiated from spells of fainting or syncope in which case there is a pallor, cold clammy skin, bradycardia), having paresthesia (feeling of "pins and needles"), severe pruritus (itching), throbbing in the ears, palpitations (rapid, pounding heart), sneezing, giant hives or generalized edema, bronchial asthma (bronchospasm with labored respiration, expiratory dyspnea with short inspirations, prolonged expirations, due to edema of the lining membranes of the respiratory tract and resulting in respiratory obstruction), wheezing, coughing, choking, stridor (laryngeal edema), cyanosis, mydriasis, hypotension, rapid, weak pulse due to hypovolemia and vasodilatation, cardiac insufficiency or arrhythmias and ventricular tachycardia, GU and GI pain and incontinence, cumulating in sudden loss of consciousness, convulsions, complete unresponsiveness, shock, respiratory depression, apnea with the patient turning ashen gray with the likely approach of death.

Immediate and vigorous therapy is life-saving: place the patient in a supine position with the legs elevated (Trendelenburg position); maintain adequate airway, employ endotracheal tube (or tracheostomy), if indicated, give positive pressure oxygen or, if not available, mouth-to-mouth resuscitation should be started (artificial ventilation). Administer epinephrine, 1:1,000 concentration, 0.3 to 1.0 ml IV; repeat injections of epinephrine in 5 to 10 minutes, if necessary. Use other vasopressor agents, e.g., norepinephrine, or phenylephrine 0.5 mg, 1%, in infusion of intravenous fluid; "plasma expanders" e.g., normal saline to cope with the arterial hypotension. Support the circulation by intravenous use of corticosteroid hormones, e.g., hydrocortisone sodium succinate (Solu-Cortef), 500 mg, IV dexamethasone (Decadron), 4 to 12 mg, this will possibly protect the "shock organs" from injury. All these maneuvers will increase venous return, cardiac output, increase stroke volume, the force of myocardial contractions and decrease antigen-antibody reactions. If cardiac arrest occurs external cardiac massage (closed chest cardiac resuscitation) must be started at once. Vital signs are monitored continuously. Antihistamines are later given, i.e., Benadryl, 50 mg IM.

Angina Pectoris and Ischemic Heart Disease

Angina pectoris is a disease condition in which myocardial ischemia occurs, usually in association with coronary artery (atherosclerotic) disease. There is a decrease of blood, therefore, oxygen, supply through one or more narrow branches of the coronary arteries.

Clinical manifestations are characteristic: sudden, severe paroxysmal precordial, substernal pain, which may radiate to the volar surface of the left arm, forearm, digitus anularis and minimus (quintus), or both arms, both shoulders, neck and the mandible. The pain is carried from the ischemic myocardium through the plexus of sympathetic nerves of the wall of coronary arteries to the spinal cord. The onset of pain is related to physical exertion, emotional disturbances, nightmares, a heavy meal, tachycardia, cold environment, recumbent position, acute hypotension and hypoglycemia. The pain is usually of short (1 to 5 minutes) duration and rarely lasts for more than 15 to 30 minutes; the patient suffers a sensation of choking, feeling of heavy squeezing, tightness, suffocation, dyspnea, vertigo, faintness and palpitations. These symptoms are present during and shortly after the attack of angina pectoris. The patient interrupts any activity in a fixed position until the attack subsides, appears ashen gray, pale, with cold sweats on the face, the respiration is superficial and there is a fear of impending death. The aftermath of the attack is usually uneventful, free from fever, circulatory collapse or shock, but the patient may be incapacitated and severely depressed following the angina. If coronary occlusion develops subsequent to the spasm of coronary arteries, the pain is intensified to a maximal level, and the patient may die during the attack. Diagnosis of this condition is made by evaluating the clinical manifestations like location of the pain concentrated at midsubstantial region, and by electrocardiogram.

In about 80% of cases the disease is predominant in aged male population having hypertensive vascular disease or organic cardiac pathology. Hypercholesterolemia or familial xanthomatosis, diabetes mellitus, obesity, myxedema, a tense business or professional life style, and smoking are the most common causes for increased susceptibility to the condition of angina pectoris. The average life span, based on international statistics, following the onset of attacks of angina pectoris is less than 16 years, maintaining the uncorrected background factors.

The treatment of an acute attack of angina pectoris should be the following:

Nitroglycerin 0.3 to 0.6 mg tablets[1] slipped under the patient's tongue (sublingually) to cause dilation of cor-

---

[1] The nitroglycerin tablets exposed to air have a short shelf life.

onary arteries (may be substituted by inhalation of crushed pearl-bud of amyl nitrite).

Place the patient in a resting (semisupine) position.

Administer oxygen (10 liter flow) via nasal canule or face mask, if necessary.

If paroxysmal tachycardia, atrial flutter or fibrillation develop, digitalis or quinidine administration should be considered.

A narcotic such as morphine 1 to 4 mg IV can be given to relieve to pain.

Sedatives such as barbiturates and laxatives may be used when absolutely necessary to provide complete physical and mental rest.

Monitor vital signs; if myocardial infarction is suspected the patient is to be transferred to the hospital emergency ward.

In reviewing the patient's medical history, think preventively prior to rendering dental services:

Provide a comfortably cool environment.

Avoid treatment after meals.

Exclude stress, anxiety and lengthy appointments.

Forbid caffeine, tobacco and alcohol prior to, during and after therapy.

Avoid hypoxia (N_2O analgesia).

Keep the suggested medicaments at hand.

Use no vasoconstrictors.

Angioneurotic Edema

It is an allergic reaction involving the skin or mucous membranes, causing swelling of subcutaneous, submucosal connective tissue areas of the eyelids, dorsum of hands and feet, genitalia, lips or lining of the larynx and upper respiratory tract, producing distress, obstruction, and a sensation of suffocation occasionally developing into life-threatening danger.

Therapeutic regimes should include epinephrine, antihistamines, and steroids and, in the case of laryngeal involvement, coniotomy should be considered.

Aortic Valvular Stenosis and Sudden Death

Aortic valvular stenosis may develop following rheumatic heart disease or infective endocarditis; it may be purely sclerotic, or may represent a congenital defect. Narrowing (stenosis) of the aortic aperture occurs due to fusion of commissural parts of semilunar valves, which may extend up to the cusp margins resulting in true aortic valvular stenosis. The distorted valve leaflets are malfunctioning, and reduction of aortic orifice will cause left ventricular hypertrophy. Physical examination should reveal sustained, slow and low pulse, holosystolic aortic murmur following the ejection click, the patient is gently flushed, with a delicate pinkish complexion, and complains of dyspnea, angina pectoris, cardiac decompensation, and oncoming syncope. These symptoms are more prominent on effort. ECG presents the picture of left ventricular hypertrophy. The treatment is usually valvotomy or valve replacement. Proper preventive precautions should include antibiotic chemoprophylaxis as described in the previous chapter.

Cardiac Arrhythmia

Emotional stress related to dental procedures can elicit alarming clinical manifestations of cardiac arrhythmias in patients having sufficiently compromised cardiovascular status, the presence of a murmur due to a damaged valve, or other organic cardiac impairment. The sign and symptoms may include irregular rate, volume and rhythm of the central or peripheral pulse, palpitations, headache, dizziness, profound weakness, dyspnea, hypotension and syncope.

Prevention of this medical complication is advised and discussed in the previous chapter.

The treatment of an episode of cardiac arrhythmia should include positioning the patient in a semisupine posture to facilitate respiration, administration of an antiarrhythmic, oxygen and narcotic analgesic. Cardiopulmonary resuscitation may be necessary.

Cardiac Arrest (Standstill) and Other Causes of Sudden Death

Ischemic heart disease.

Hypertensive vascular disease (MI, CVA).

Valvular stenosis/insufficiency.

Congenital heart disease.

1° pulmonary hypertension.

Ruptured cerebral aneurysm.
Anaphylaxis, electric shock.
Acute fulminant infections.
Asphyxia

SIGNS AND SYMPTOMS

  a. Feeling of apprehension.
  b. Shortness of breath.
  c. Severe pain, usually described as a crushing pressure beneath the breast bone. The pain may appear first in the left arm, radiate into the neck, and then to the left side of the chest.
  d. Nausea and vomiting.
  e. Sweating.
  f. Cyanosis.
  g. Unconsciousness/dilation of pupils.
  h. Absence of pulse and heart sounds, blood pressure is not measurable, apnea and agonal gasping (respiration by using the accessory muscles).
  i. In case of open surgery the blood appears dark, followed by cessation of hemorrhage.

Clinical death in 4 to 5 minutes, biologic death (irreversible) in about 8 minutes.

TREATMENT

  a. Place the patient in a sitting position (or if the patient is unconscious, in a supine position with the neck extended).
  b. Apply oxygen under positive pressure after assuring an adequate airway.
  c. Do not allow the patient to assist in moving himself.
  d. Comfort and reassure the patient.
  e. Loosen the clothing.
  f. If necessary, give cardiopulmonary resuscitation (40% success in an intensive care unit, 10% survival in an office environment).
  g. Seek immediate medical attention.

Cardiac Decompensation

Cardiac decompensation, congestive heart failure, occurs when the ability of the heart to function as demanded over a prolonged period exceeds what is called the cardiac reserve. Generally in cardiovascular disease, as seen in patients with high arterial blood pressure, arteriosclerotic heart disease, this cardiac reserve diminishes gradually until the heart is no longer able to sufficiently fulfill the normal physiologic demands, to circulate the quantities of blood required because of degenerative changes in the myocardium, or the demand on the damaged heart is increased by a higher metabolic rate, or there is an insufficient venous return to the heart.

The clinical manifestations of congestive heart failure are related to the insufficient cardiac output, inefficient blood supply to vital organs and accumulation of connective tissue fluid in the liver, the lungs, kidneys and brain, depending on the degree of severity of the disease. Signs and symptoms would include shortness of breath upon moderate exercise, progressing into dyspnea at rest, orthopnea (resting in sitting position, sleeping on two or more pillows) with labored breathing, chronic cough with blood stained sputum due to pulmonary congestion, general fatigue, chest pain, dependent edema such as ankle swelling (anasarca), some degree of mydriasis, rapid weak pulse, cyanosis of the lips, oral mucosa, and the tongue, distension of lingual ranine veins and neck veins.

These cardiac patients are usually on medications such as digitalis and diuretics. The dental appointments should be short, in the morning when the patient is not very fatigued, maintaining a comfortable sitting position at room temperature. The patient should receive calm reassuring management, restriction of any physical efforts, and quiet, quick and efficient dental procedures. Administration of morphine, a sedative, or oxygen should be considered. Extensive elective dental treatment is unnecessary. Procedures should be limited to one quadrant per appointment under skillfully applied local anesthesia; frequent routine recall visits should be scheduled.

Cardiopulmonary Resuscitation

In case of cardiac arrest due to cardiovascular collapse (weak systole without measurable blood pressure and perceptible pulse), ventricular fibrillation (irregular contractions of myocardial syncytium without blood flow through the arteries), ventricular standstill (asystole—no heartbeat) and respiratory arrest indicate the need for cardiopulmonary resuscitation

(CPR) by employing the basic life support immediately in rapid, automatic succession:

   a. *Airway* restoration and maintenance.

   b. *Breathing* restoration by artificial ventilation and maintenance with delivery of oxygen.

   c. *Circulation* restoration by artificial circulation and maintenance.

   d. *Drug* administration.

Remember: following pupillary dilatation there are about 2 minutes left for CPR.

The respiration should first be restored to avoid blood circulation with low oxygen as well as high carbon dioxide concentrations.

To prevent unnecessary CPR and cause possible damage to both respiratory and circulatory systems in "deep sleepers" or fainters, the victim should be shaken and asked loudly, "Hey, how are you, are you all right?"

a. *Airway* (and breathing) restoration is the basic step of artificial ventilation. Respiratory failure or arrest is characterized by the absence of respiratory movement (chest, abdomen), no air movement is detected through the mouth and nose (use a mirror), or labored breathing is present from airway obliteration, and resulting in respiratory insufficiency. Opening of the airways is an immediate act by tilting back the patient's head with one hand placed on the forehead, the other at the back of the neck lifting up and expanding the neck, while the tongue is forced forward to open up the pharynx. Clear the air passage, if necessary. This position should be maintained effectively to secure successful resuscitation. Observe for breathing.

b. *Breathing*, if absent, is restored by starting artificial ventilation through mouth-to-mouth, or mouth-to-nose, or mouth-to-airway. For effective mouth-to-mouth ventilation the nostrils of the patient should be pinched off with the same hand pressing the forehead, taking a deep inspiration, make an airtight seal around the mouth of the victim and blow until the chest of the patient expands well, then let the victim exhale while watching closely the expiratory movement of the chest. Inflate lungs by four initial quick breaths. Repeat this cycle once every 4 to 5 seconds until adequate spontaneous respiration is resumed. For infants or young children, less back tilt of the head and milder neck extension are recommended in order to avoid airway obliteration. Less air volume should be used and repeated once every 3 seconds.

Mouth-to-nose ventilation may be preferred by the rescuer, the mouth area may be seriously injured, it may be impossible to open the patient's mouth, or difficult to achieve a tight seal around the lips. In this technique the mandible is forced into occlusion and the lips are sealed with the hand otherwise used to lift the back of the neck. Care must be taken to separate the lips and open the mouth to let the air escape during expiration since the soft palate may separate the nasopharynx from the oropharynx.

If a foreign body (vomitus, blood, teeth) obstructs the upper respiratory air passages it should be removed by the fingers, or forceps. If the foreign object cannot be dislodged this way the patient should be rolled on one side facing the rescuer, or a small patient may be picked up and inverted over the arm or shoulder of the rescuer, who would forcefully bang the patient's back between the scapulae or perform the Heimlich maneuver and repeat attempted artificial ventilation. If still not possible, try to eliminate the artifact again and consider coniotomy.

c. *Circulation.* Immediately following four quick lung inflations if cardiac arrest is present (absence of central pulse and heart sounds, mydriasis), artificial circulation is indicated via external cardiac compressions. While maintaining the artificial ventilation the patient is placed on a hard surface in Trendelenburg's position (autotransfusion) to facilitate cerebral circulation. Place the heel of one hand over the lower half of the sternum (not over the xiphoid process, to prevent liver laceration), position the other hand on top of the first one, and with straight arms apply enough pressure to compress the sternum 5 to 6 cm towards the vertebral column.

If the rescuer is afraid to fracture some ribs the logical question should be raised: "Is an alive patient with broken ribs better than an intact dead victim?" The compressions should be intermittent, regular and smooth, equal in duration to allow diastolic cardiac filling, but strong enough to compress the heart and force the blood out of the ventricles. The rhythmic compression rate is one per second to maintain adequate blood flow, and must be combined with the artificial ventilation interposed after each five compressions, for example:

1 operator: 15 compressions/2 inflations (rate is 80 compressions per minute).

2 operators: 5 compressions/1 inflation (rate is 60 compressions per minute).

To avoid fatigue there is an allowance for fifteen chest compressions followed by two full but quick lung inflations (to achieve the 60 per minute heart compressions in spite of lung inflations the rate of cardiac compressions must be increased to 80 per minute). Infants and young children receive milder compressions delivered to the middle of the sternum by the tips of digitus index and medius and the heel of one hand, to depress the sternum 1.5 to 2 cm, or 2 to 3 cm, respectively, at a compression rate of 80 to 100 per minute intermingled with one ventilation after two compressions. The abdomen must be palpated and compressed if the stomach becomes inflated with air.

In complete cardiac arrest (the carotid pulse and cardiac sounds are absent), or to reverse certain dysrhythmias (ventricular tachycardia), precordial thump may be effective to start normal cardiac rhythm. The precordial thump is a strong, quick, single blow delivered by the fist over the mid-portion of the sternum. In the absence of an immediate circulatory response start the CPR at once. If the CPR is successful the dilated pupils begin to constrict, the cyanosis (stasis and reduced hemoglobin) will decrease, there is an attempted return of spontaneous respiratory movement, and the patient's normal pulse rhythm becomes detectable; purposeful bodily movements occur.

Laryngeal intubation, available in infant, child and adult sizes, may be used if the patient is unconscious (may cause vomiting and laryngospasm in a conscious patient). There are air bag-valve mask devices and S-tubes to facilitate the airtight seal during artificial ventilation.

Oxygen equipment (rate of O_2 flow should be 10 liters per minute) is effective to provide successful artificial ventilation and reduce hypoxia of the brain, since the expired air can give 14 to 17% oxygen to the victim.

A defibrillator is often effective (no pulse, mydriasis) in correcting ventricular fibrillation and restoring the normal cardiac cycle. Deliver a single electric shock by the defibrillator: one electrode is placed on the left of the right nipple, the other is next to the left lateral chest. (An ECG should monitor the cardiac status during this procedure.)

d. *Drugs* should be utilized to secure the success of CPR (if the patient is pulseless and has mydriasis 5 minutes after the start of CPR), including epinephrine, in 1:1,000 concentration, 0.5 ml IV, or intratracheal (1.5 mg per 9 ml saline), or intracardiac, repeated every 5 minutes, during the resuscitation to start the arrested heart. It helps restore the normal sinus rhythm and increases myocardiac contractility. If weak carotid pulse is palpated give phenylephrine (Neo-Synephrine), 1:500, 1 ml, IV (2 mg); or ephedrine, 25 to 50 mg; or levarterenol (Levophed), 0.5 mg; or isoproterenol, 45 mg. Sodium bicarbonate, 10 ml of 3.75 gm per 50 ml sol. IV every 5 minutes, is given to compensate for elevated levels of lactic acid in the hypoxic tissues—the metabolic acidosis. Atropine sulfate, 0.6 mg IV (total dose not to exceed 2 mg), should be given if systolic blood pressure is below 90 mm Hg and pulse rate is less than 60 per minute, repeated every 5 minutes until the normal sinus rhythm is reached, to accelerate heart rate in sinus bradycardia, enhance A-V (atrioventricular) conduction and reduce vagal tone. Lidocaine, 50 to 100 mg IV is effective to raise the fibrillation threshold (of no value in asystole). Calcium chloride will enhance ventricular excitability, prolong systole and increase myocardial contractility. Morphine sulfate is contraindicated in CPR (it is useful in MI to relieve pain). The drug administrations should not interrupt the CPR and should be given with medical supervision. Monitor vital signs, record patient responses and drugs administered.

The CPR should be continued uninterrupted until effective spontaneous respiration and circulation are restored, or the patient is transferred to assure continuing care to maintain the basic life support of the victim. Transfer the patient quickly to the hospital emergency ward.

CONIOTOMY

Coniotomy (cricothyroid membrane incision or "tracheostomy") is indicated when the airway is obturated above the vocal cords and no attempt to dislodge the blockage (Heimlich maneuver = firm abdominal pressure) is efficient in removing that obstruction. If the obstruction is located inferior to the conic ligament, a tracheotomy (tracheostomy) should be performed as follows.

Place the patient in the Trendelenburg position.

Hyperextend the neck (head and neck are in the midsagittal plane of the body).

Make a 20-mm transverse skin incision over the conic ligament (between the inferior margin of the thyroid cartilage and the superior margin of the cricoid cartilage) and open the wound by stretching the skin with the index and middle fingers.

Puncture the conic ligament with a small sharp scissors, insert the beaks into the lumen of the airway.

Dilate the conic ligament transversely by expanding the beaks.

Introduce a tube (minimum 10 mm inside diameter) between the beaks of the scissors through the opening on the conic ligament and remove the scissors.

Secure the tube (surgical tape) into place and transfer the patient to the hospital emergency ward for radiographs (posteroanterior and lateral chest view, bronchoscopy, abdominal flat plane x-ray, if indicated).

Note: if the procedure is done with nonsterile materials (e.g., a pocket knife) the patient should receive antibiotics in the hospital.

Dissecting Aneurysm (Aneurysm of the Abdominal Aorta)

Dissecting aneurysm is the condition of intramural hemorrhage into the media of a large blood vessel, involving, most frequently, the aorta, commonly around 40 years of age. The absence of inflammation is characteristic, there is fatty, hyaline or mucoid degeneration of the connective tissue components, atrophy of the smooth muscle fibers and fragmentation of elastic fibers in the vessel walls. Hypothyroidism, hypertension, Morgan's syndrome with coarctation of the aorta and sometimes pregnancy is pointed out as an etiologic factor. The direct cause, as believed by most pathologists, is the extravasation of blood from a ruptured vasa vasorum into the media initiated by a sudden increase in blood pressure due to physical or psychological stress, or, rarely, the complication of carotid arteriography. About 70% of dissecting aneurysms begin in the ascending aorta, 1 to 2 cm above the aortic orifice. Dissecting aneurysm may result in perforation through the outer portion of the wall into the pericardial cavity (cardiac tamponade), producing sudden death; or may dissect along the intramural portion proximally, obliterating the coronary orifices and leading to aortic valvular insufficiency; or distally into the origin of the branching large arteries causing obstruction of their lumen; or may rupture back to the aortic lumen through a secondary reentry penetration of the intima, in which case thrombosis, organization and fibrous obliteration can result in spontaneous cure of the condition.

In a typical attack there is a usually severe thoracic pain radiating to the neck, head and back area, lasting perhaps for several hours, causing dyspnea and profound emotional distress, hypertension, weakness and paralysis of the extremities resulting in hemiplegia, hematemesis, hematuria, congestive cardiac decompensation and syncope.

Epileptic Seizures

In about 85% of seizure patients reverberating electric currents of the cerebrum can be recorded by EEG during epileptic seizures which may be related to organic brain lesions (symptomatic epilepsy), such as degenerative, inflammatory processes, meningitis, encephalitis, brain abscess, vascular lesions, birth and other trauma, insulin hypoglycemia, drug (alcohol) intoxication, neoplasm, fluid and electrolyte disorder, neurologic (migraine) disturbances, heredity, but often no organic or pathophysiologic cause can be detected (idiopathic epilepsy). Most seizures occurring before the age of twenty are idiopathic.

CLINICAL MANIFESTATIONS

a. Status epilepticus: a series of grand mal seizures with unconsciousness.

b. Grand mal epilepsy: a short period of aura is present in 50% of cases, including visual disturbances (flash of light), headache, strange smell, taste, sound, abnormal visceral sensation, apathy, depression, irritability, sensation of alertness and ecstasy, bizarre thoughts; then there is a moan or cry (caused by contraction of the diaphragm and chest muscles), paleness, tingling of lips or fingers, loss of consciousness, fall to the ground, involuntary tonic-clonic spasms of the skeletal musculature and autonomic nervous system disturbances resulting in visceral activity, urinary and fecal incontinence, tongue biting, contortion of the face, eyes rolled up or to the side; cuts, bruises and fractures are common. Sialorrhea, sweating, mydriasis, cyanosis (due to interference with respiration) and hypertension, tachypnea, tachycardia are present. The usual duration of the attack is a few (3 to 4) minutes, the frequency varies up to several per day. Following the seizure there is amnesia, confusion, drowsiness, headache and muscle pains.

c. Jacksonian seizures: fixes eyes, paresthesia begins at the distal part of one extremity, spreads centrally and is followed by clonic convulsive movements which may involve the entire body, developing into a grand mal convulsion with loss of consciousness and coma. The attacks usually follow the same clinical pattern each time.

d. Petit mal epilepsy is characterized by momentary clouding of consciousness or transient unconsciousness and paleness. Usually associated with minor muscle contractions (twitching) of the eyelids, head or extremities, the loss of muscle tone may result in a fall to the ground, the sudden interruption of activity performed, fixed posture and vertigo. The attack may last for several seconds and occur many times

a day. When any seizure occurs one must rule out seizures caused by hypoglycemia, vasovagal syncope, cerebrovascular accident or drugs.

Management of an epileptic condition should begin with preventive measures, including medications such as diphenyl-hydantoin-Na (Dilantin), phenobarbital, Tridione, etc. The dose, the drug of choice and the frequency of administration depend on the type and severity of epilepsy; other preventive measures include the avoidance of excitement leading to seizures, e.g., anesthetics containing epinephrine or nitrous oxide analgesia, and the avoidance of alcohol consumption and vehicle driving where indicated.

In case of a pending seizure, maintain a patent airway, eliminate removable prosthetic appliances to prevent their dislodgement or aspiration, oxygen should be given (it is wise to deliver oxygen for any phase and at an early stage of epileptic seizure to prevent cerebral hypoxia and brain damage).

Patient management during a convulsive seizure is directed toward avoiding damage to the patient or the environment. Place the patient on the ground away from all the solid objects, place a soft pad under the head and hold the extremities away from objects, prevent tongue and lip injuries, or fracture of the teeth, or the luxation of the mandible by using a rolled towel, a rubber mouth prop or well padded tongue blade between the teeth. Tight clothing should be loosened, insuring proper ventilation; oxygen should be administered by oral or nasal mask with maintenance of a good airway. Dilantin may be given at a rate of 50 mg every minute up to 1 gram or until convulsions cease. If Dilantin fails to control the seizure phenobarbital or Valium is indicated. Although death may commence during status epilepticus, the prognosis is usually not grave. Unless pronounced mental deterioration or severe injury occurs the outlook is good and the patient may function as a normal member of society.

Extrapyramidal Reactions

Extrapyramidal reactions include the sudden onset of involuntary tongue movements, contractions of masticatory muscles, bizarre facial expressions, prolonged contractions of cervical muscles (usually unilateral, intermittent), tardive dyskinesia (flapping or "fly catching" tongue movements, sucking lips, masticatory movements) or akathisia (persistent, or repetitive motion), often related to the intake of phenothiazine tranquilizers (antipsychotic medications), provided the patient does not have underlying disease of the extrapyramidal system, i.e., Parkinsonism.

Administration of diphenhydramine-HCl (Benadryl) up to 50 mg IM is suggested in an emergency situation.

Foreign Body Aspiration (Asphyxia)

When a foreign material passes the oropharynx, as in normal deglutition, it enters the esophagus, passes through the gastrointestinal tract and may cause no complications (i.e., a lost crown can be recovered in about 3 days). If the foreign object is aspirated and lodged in the larynx, trachea or tracheobronchial tree the patient will exhibit manifestations of acute respiratory obstruction. A minor foreign body impaction at the level of the glottal opening produces a choking sensation, partial laryngospasm and forceful coughing, and often results in successful expelling of the foreign body. More significant obstruction will elicit gasping for air, coughing, gagging in an attempt to expel the foreign object, straining of neck and chest muscles, severe restlessness with aphonia or high pitched whistling tones, stridor (harsh, vibrating), and the skin turns cyanotic. Complete laryngospasm may prevent sufficient alveolar respiration, and the victim passes into unconsciousness.

In order to prevent this emergency situation during dental treatment such as nitrous oxide analgesia, general anesthesia, local anesthetic procedures, endodontic treatment or prosthetic impressions, etc., the rubber dam, where indicated, and care should be employed.

If an object is lost in the mouth, the patient should open the mouth, refrain from deglutition as well as deep inspiration. Instruct the patient to breathe via the nose, until the recovery of the foreign object from the pharynx is achieved by grasping and pulling the tongue forward and cleaning the pharynx with instruments, suction or fingers. If the foreign object has entered the respiratory tract and caused obstruction at the level of the vocal cords or above the cricoid cartilage, a quick emergency coniotomy should be performed by using a 13 gauge needle at the midline raphe through the cricothyroid (conic) ligament, (see Coniotomy). If the foreign body obturated the distal segment of the trachea, use tracheostomy. The tracheostomy, which involves section of a tracheal cartilage, may require ligation of the thyroid isthmus. Adequate ventilation should be supported with oxygen administration or artificial respiration.

Hyperglycemic (Diabetic) Coma

In patients with uncontrolled diabetes mellitus the insufficient insulin supply and the consequent increase of glucose levels in the blood circulation, as well as in the tissues of the body, can result in unconsciousness and coma. This danger requires carefully matched insulin-diet regime.

Hyperglycemic coma condition is most often elicited by the dramatic reduction or the complete omission of the administration of proper insulin dose (or other prescribed antidiabetic medication). The frequent reasons are that the patient:

Forgets to inject the insulin or take the oral agent.

Becomes seriously ill and unable to administer the drug.

Is on oral antidiabetic medication and experiences drug interaction (alcohol, chlorthalidone, corticosteroids, epinephrine, isoniazid, thiazides).

Stops the administration of antidiabetic medication since he is feeling well and misbelieves that he has become cured.

Takes diet pills, loses weight and appetite and consequently stops taking the antidiabetic medication.

Many times horrible hyperphagia (excessive food consumption), acute generalized intercurrent, or severe exacerbation of systemic illness is detected as interfering with the delicate control of diabetes mellitus. Since about 25% of diabetic cases are unrecognized (in spite of the presence of clinical manifestations) it is possible to see these patients present with diabetic coma.

The clinical manifestations of hyperglycemic coma develop relatively slowly during several days, the patient feels extremely ill, exhibiting the cardinal signs (polyphagia, polyuria, particularly nocturia, polydipsia); a craving for sweet beverages, thirst is intensive, and the mouth is progressively dry (xerostomia). Other symptoms include excessive tiredness, drowsiness, malaise, lassitude, loss of appetite and weight, nausea, vomitus and generalized abdominal pain; hyperventilation (forceful, deep sighings); noticeable acetone odor of the breath due to production of ketones (gluconeogenesis with protein and fat catabolism at a dangerous level, diabetic acidosis); dehydration (the skin appears to be inelastic, wrinkled, dry, flushed, red, warm); the ocular tone is decreased and the lens capsule is corrugated, giving the impression of cataracts; fever, vertigo, restlessness, mental confusion; and, as circulatory collapse commences, hypotension, weak rapid pulse (tachycardia), loss of consciousness and hypothermia terminating in coma.

In the case of an impending coma place the patient in a supine position, administer oxygen and keep the patient warm (blanket).

To gain time for blood glucose determination (Dextrostix) and to diagnose the presence of diabetic coma start the emergency treatment with 5% dextrose in normal saline IV. Record vital signs. If the diagnosis is established, administer insulin in IV infusion line. (Remember, the transport of insulin is rapid out of the blood circulation: 4 minutes half-life. Therefore, if the continuous IV infusion is not possible, insulin is given IM every hour till the diabetic coma is suppressed.) Improvement is slow, beginning in 6 to 12 hours, but by that time the patient should be transferred to the hospital emergency ward. The cardiovascular collapse and severe dehydration (vomitus) require IV fluid and electrolyte replacement and possibly vasoconstrictors.

Hyperventilation

Hyperventilation syndrome of psychogenic origin is usually the result of acute anxiety, fear, stress (release of epinephrine) manifesting most commonly in tense, nervous female patients with profound emotional disturbances and underlying sympathetic overtone. The hyperventilation causes hypocapnia (excess elimination of carbon dioxide) and respiratory alkalosis. The early clinical signs and symptoms would include abnormally deep, rapid respiration for a prolonged period, a sensation of tightness in the chest, a feeling of suffocation, excessive deep sighs, severe apprehension, lightheadedness, nausea, sialorrhea, sweating, paleness, impaired consciousness, paresthesia, cold extremities and perioral areas, muscle cramps, spasms which may develop into tetany, precordial pressure pain, epigastric distress, generalized discomfort, palpitations, blurred vision, sensation of decreased awareness, faintness, yawning, and later, as the abnormal deep respiration (hyperpnea) continues, the further decrease of CO_2 partial pressure initiates peripheral vasodilatation, hypotension and actual syncope with pupillary dilatation, bradycardia and often convulsive movements.

When this condition occurs the breath-holding, a paper bag or reservoir rebreathing bag (to limit the eliminated amount of CO_2), along with reassurance, is often sufficient to correct the syndrome. A supine position will efficiently postpone the development of unconsciousness in severe cases. Sedation may be indicated.

An attack may last for an hour and may recur at any time with unpredictable frequency. The patient often suffers severe headache, and is confused and weak on recovery.

The treatment should include, in case of syncope, the autotransfusion (recumbent position, elevation of the legs) and O_2 administration to cope with cerebral hypoxia.

Hypoglycemic Coma (Insulin Shock or Reaction)

Hypoglycemia is one of the most common diagnoses in cases of unconscious, unknown patients. The condition can develop for several reasons:

Extreme dietary restrictions (insufficient or delayed meals with no carbohydrate intake, starvation).

Unusually heavy and prolonged physical exercise.

Voluminous vomiting periods, protracted diarrhea.

In diagnosed diabetics the hypoglycemia can be induced:

By inadvertent IV injection of insulin.

By insulin overdose (insulin reaction or shock) or oral antidiabetic medication).

If the patient is on oral antidiabetic medication (the sulfonylurea derivatives) and experiences drug interaction (sulfonamides, acetylsalicylic acid).

During the initial phase of oral antidiabetic management when the control of food intake (obesity) is prescribed.

The patient is on oral antidiabetic medication and has adrenal, pituitary or hepatic disease.

In extreme cases when the dose of antidiabetic medication is elevated at the onset of menstruation and not reduced for the postmenstrual stage.

If the dose of insulin injection is calibrated at a cold temperature, the patient moves to a hot environment (a hot environment decreases the insulin demand) and keeps receiving the same insulin dose.

The clinical manifestations of hypoglycemia vary with different levels of blood glucose, individual response of patient, time of onset and type of insulin used (sudden onset if regular soluble insulin is injected, slow onset if long-acting insulin is administered and the intermediate is in between; this is especially prominent if the elimination of postprandial glucosuria is attempted during the early stage of patient management).

The onset signs and symptoms of hypoglycemia commence within hours: restlessness, irritability, nervousness, anxiety, intense hunger, weakness, drowsiness, headache, dizziness, diplopia, vertigo, inability to concentrate, mental confusion, aphasia, unsteadiness, incoordination, muscle twitching, trembling, staggering gait, ataxia, sometimes vomiting, sialorrhea, paresthesia of the extremities, tingling sensation of oral and perioral structures, pallor, early, full bounding pulse, increased perspiration, faintness, progressive development of circulatory collapse;

profound hypotension, cold, clammy skin (mainly extremities), loss of consciousness, actual convulsions, stupor and coma.

Prevention includes detection of patients having diabetes mellitus, taking a thorough health history, evaluation of the level of control of the diabetic patient at each appointment to make sure that the patient has taken the usual insulin dosage, and has also eaten sufficient calories to be metabolized by the insulin (or oral antihyperglycemic agent). Keeping dental appointments within reasonable time limits to avoid fasting for hours, exhausting the absorbed carbohydrate and failing to supply sufficient nourishment at the proper time; avoidance of dental services in the risk patient with intercurrent febrile or other serious systemic illness; determining the level of control (blood/urine glucose) prior to stressful, extensive dental procedures; checking on the careful matching of insulin dosages and balanced metabolism of sufficient calories; averting an impending hypoglycemic attack by the administration of sugar (sugar reinforced orange juice, 2 teaspoons of sugar, candy), usually results in recovery in 10 minutes, or a further 20 gm of carbohydrate are to be given. If the patient cannot swallow or is unconscious 50 ml of 50% glucose IV should be given, or injection of glucagon may be administered. Subcutaneous injection of 0.5 to 1.0 ml (1:1,000 concentration) epinephrine raises rapidly and temporarily the blood glucose level with quick improvement.

If the existence of insulin shock or diabetic coma is undetermined and the patient does not respond to administration of oxygen or a broken capsule of spirits of ammonia, the 5% dextrose IV or 50 ml of 50% glucose IV is indicated without delay to prevent permanent brain damage (developing in 5 minutes in severe hypoglycemia). Upon recovery the relapse can be prevented by giving a further 30 gm of carbohydrate orally. Severe headache with retrograde amnesia may point to a serious degree of cerebral hypoglycemia.

Laryngospasm

Spastic reflex, partial or complete contraction of intralaryngeal muscles, and vocal cord adduction by the intrinsic muscles may be induced by the sudden inhalation of high concentrations of the N_2O analgesic, general anesthetic, administration of an IV barbiturate, parasympathomimetic agents, irritation caused by blood, mucus or aspiration of foreign material (polluted air, dust, heavy smoking) is most commonly seen if the patient suffers from chronic bronchitis, emphysema, bronchiectasis, chronic pulmonary disease and central nervous system depression. The signs and symptoms of stridor, cough, respiratory depression, dyspnea and apnea, hypoxia or anoxia with cyanosis and progressive onset of circulatory depression terminating in cardiac arrest may be witnessed in minutes.

Prevention of this emergency situation prior to nitrous analgesia, inhalation anesthesia is the effective premedication with atropine or scopolamine (parasympatholytic agents to block mucous production of pharynx, larynx, the irritation of the vocal cords and initiation of laryngospasm). Prevention of dyspnea by insurance of sufficient oxygenation, proper patient positioning, the use of a rubber dam or oropharyngeal packing are important steps in preventive patient management.

The actual treatment of laryngospasm consists of 10 to 20 mg Anectine (succinylcholine), IV to relax the laryngeal muscles (the muscle relaxation interrupts the reflex anatomic blockade elicited by the irritating substance). If the possible danger of aspiration is absent, and a tonsil suction tip is available to remove secretions from the pharynx (the tongue is promoted), administer positive pressure 100% oxygen through an adequate airway or administer frank artificial ventilation, if necessary, by using a full facial (or nasal) mask, respiratory bag (or mouth-to-mouth, mouth-to-nose technique) since succinylcholine will paralyze respiratory muscles. To reestablish patent air passages the coniotomy procedure may be necessary (see Coniotomy).

Myocardial Infarction

Sudden occlusion of a coronary artery or sufficiently long-lasting interference with the blood flow through a branch of the coronary artery—perhaps due to embolism or thrombosis—can cause myocardial ischemia and subsequent tissue necrosis, depending on the delivery capacity of the collateral blood circulation.

Myocardial infarction is most common in the 40- to 50-year-old male who smokes and is a stressed, highly strained worker with intense worries. Frequently he has a history of angina pectoris, hypertensive vascular disease, arteriosclerosis, diabetes, with or without associated warning signs and symptoms, or physical exercise, emotional distress, excitement. Myocardial infarction often occurs at rest or during sleep.

Clinical manifestations are characterized by extreme fear, intense squeezing pressure, pain localized at the precordial, midsternal area, often radiating to the left arm or mandible similar to angina pectoris, usually persisting for hours. Certain patients may develop a fatal complication of shock syndrome (inadequate perfusion of blood to vital organs), cardiac arrhythmias, cold perspiration, restlessness, nausea, vomiting, weakness, cardiac decompensation, progressive hypotension, decreased pulse pressure, thready pulse, cyanosis, tachyarrhythmia and later bradyarrhythmia, pulmonary edema, faintness, mental confusion and peripheral circulatory collapse. The chest pain is not relieved by nitroglycerin tablets. ECG presents changes which occur in more than 80%. Polymorphonuclear leukocytosis is present on the second day, and enzyme changes may permit definite diagnosis.

If the acute myocardial infarct is not immediately fatal, there is a good chance to survive; some patients may suffer several myocardial infarcts. Since dental treatment can precipitate this emergency condition a thorough medical history, e.g., prothrombin time if the patient is on anticoagulant therapy, and evaluation of cardiac status should be completed before rendering the dental services, combined with good pain control, premedication, and nontraumatic techniques to be performed with minimal appointment time. Elective dental therapy is contraindicated during the convalescent period.

The emergency management of an acute attack should include maintenance of open airways, and continuous administration of

100% oxygen. The dentist should allay apprehension and pain (Demerol 25 to 75 mg, IM, or morphine sulfate 3 to 4 mg IV), position the victim in a comfortable semi-supine posture, give quiet reassurance, and, if shock develops, lower the head, keep the patient warm and monitor vital signs. Consider fluids and norepinephrine to increase arterial pressure without causing aggravation of ischemic status; consider atropine sulfate (0.6 mg, IV) if bradycardia should occur and a patent IV with 5% dextrose in saline should be started. Keep the patient under constant supervision, assure "comfort" and immediately transfer him to a hospital.

If cardiac arrest should develop (sudden unconsciousness, cardiac as well as respiratory standstill) apply CPR immediately as described earlier.

Narcotic Overdose

Narcotic drugs—including the opium derivatives morphine and codeine—may produce characteristic dose related clinical signs and symptoms, including drowsiness, headache, difficult concentration, lurid fantasies, giddiness, euphoria, dysphoria, slow mental functions and disorientation in time and space, relative indifference to distressing painful stimulation or complete analgesia, flushing, skin exanthems, a transient sensation of nausea and vomiting, urinary retention, constipation, miosis, sedation and the gradual onset of reversible unconsciousness from which the patient at first may be aroused (mild intoxication). The severe overdose is characterized by stupor, deep narcosis, coma, with irregular respiration (tachypnea with apnea, Cheyne-Stokes), cyanosis, tachycardia, muscle relaxation, areflexia, progressive fall in blood pressure, hypotension, the onset of bradycardia with feeble pulse, hypothermia, paleness, cold perspiration, and respiratory depression terminating in complete apnea.

If addiction or physical dependence develops, the victim attempts to regain routinely the state of euphoria by administration of increasingly larger doses of the narcotic, with progressively transient success. In this tolerant state there is a gross craving for the narcotic drug in addicts, restlessness, agitation, anxiety, anorexia with weight loss, extensive perspiration with piloerectal muscle contractions (gooseflesh), rhinorrhea, lacrimation, frequent yawning, muscle aches, cramps, twitching, mydriasis, abdominal distress, nausea, vomiting, diarrhea, insomnia, hypertension and tachycardia. The treatment of narcotic intoxication depends on the severity of the overdose, including administration of narcotic antagonists to prevent, reduce or abolish the severe CNS depressant effect of the narcotic drug. These agents can be used interchangeably, and including levallorphan (Lorfan), 1 mg IV or nalorphine (Nalline) 10 mg IV, or naloxone (Narcan), 0.4 mg, 1 ml, IM, IV. and may be repeated, if necessary, in 10 to 15 minutes, since the duration of action of narcotic antagonist is less than that of the narcotic drug.

Administration of oxygen and application of external heat to maintain normal temperature are required.

If the emergency drug overdose treatment is successful, with respiration and circulation adequately restored, the recovery may be associated with the distressing signs and symptoms of withdrawal. It is customary to substitute the opiate with a synthetic narcotic drug, e.g., methadone, by reducing its dose and executing final abrupt withdrawal, or instituting a slow reduction (over several days) of doses of the addicted drug which may result in only a mild, though more protracted, abstinence syndrome. Such a course should be supported by psychotherapy, supervised drug administration and extensive care with post-treatment guidance.

Pulmonary Valvular Stenosis and Sudden Death

In this condition there is an insufficient pulmonary blood supply. Auscultation can reveal prominent ejection click, loud holosystolic murmur at the pulmonary semilunar valves.

In mild to moderate involvement, in addition, wide splitting of the second heart sound is present, ECG changes of the right ventricular hypertrophy and right atrial dilatation (similar to the findings of pulmonary hypertension and thromboembolism) are seen. The left ventricular output is decreased. The patient is relatively active and is in moderate comfort. In severe pulmonary stenosis pronounced dyspnea, generalized asthenia, angina pectoris, cyanosis, weak and small pulse are seen with pending syncope. These patients represent extreme risk for dental treatment, often have a history of open heart surgery (valvotomy), require antibiotic chemoprophylaxis and can rapidly develop cardiovascular complications with fatal termination.

Ruptured Abdominal Aortic Aneurysm

Aneurysm, an arteriolar dilatation, is most likely initiated by the decrease, or loss of elastic capacity of the blood vessel walls (arterioles, arteries, aorta), resulting in early fusiform dilation, as well as tortuosity of these vessels. Secondary aneurysms are most frequent in arteriosclerosis; syphilis represents 5 to 10% of the causes. Progressive dilation may develop with the loss of structural integrity and partial internal rupture of the vessel wall, resulting in sacculation of the aneurysm: this saccule is usually filled with a laminated clot that may throw emboli into the blood circulation, or be the source of a superimposed bacterial infection.

Aneurysm of the abdominal aorta is most common in men after 50 years of age. These patients may present with prominent abdominal aortic pulsation, a tender abdominal (epigastric or retroumbilical) mass expanding relatively rapidly, with or without dull back pain or midabdominal persistent or intermittent pain associated with pulsation.

High arterial blood pressure is a common complicating factor. If the aneurysm and rupture involve the thoracic aorta the prognosis is grave.

Minor retroperitoneal hemorrhages from a small initial aneurysm may produce severe backaches. The severely intense pain indicates a rapidly enlarging aneurysm or major rupture. Fever, peritonitis, pneumonia, leukocytosis and moderate blood loss are within the clinical diagnostic scope. Transport the patient quickly to the hospital.

Ruptured Cerebral Aneurysm and Sudden Death

The most common site of the berry aneurysm is the circle of Willis. The patient develops signs and symptoms of sudden and extremely grave headache, enormous prostration, exhaustion, vertigo, vomiting, restlessness, irritability, drowsiness, delirium, sudden unconsciousness, collapse, convulsions with resultant coma and decerebrate rigidity; death may occur without hours. If the patient survives, bed rest, adequate food and fluid intake are to be provided. Neurosurgery may save the life of the victim.

Serum Sickness

An allergic type of reaction is commonly present a week after administration of serum to a sensitized patient. The clinical manifestations are urticaria, skin exanthems, macular "pimples" or papules, large scarlatiniform red eruptions, pruritus, lymphadenopathy (usually regional, but may be generalized), fever, splenomegaly, arthralgias and polyarthritis with periarticular inflammatory edema.

Symptomatic treatment is given to relieve pruritus by adequate doses of oral antihistamines, the arthralgia is palliated by salicylates (aspirin), or in more involved cases by cortisone administration. The drug administration can be discontinued when the signs and symptoms of serum sickness disappear.

Shock (Hypoperfusion Syndrome or Hypovolemic Shock)

Most commonly the shock is due to acute hemorrhage, which occurs in the case of accidental trauma such as burns that are large enough to decrease the circulating blood volume and result in severe hypovolemia. The loss of formed elements of the blood circulation, the plasma fluids and the electrolytes can be either extra- or intracorporeal (into the relatively inaccessible pleural or peritoneal cavities—"the third compartments"—or the lumen of the gastrointestinal and genitourinary systems). Anaphylaxis, cardiac decompensation, sepsis or dehydration may produce the same clinical manifestations of shock. Concomitant surgical blood loss, dehydration, poor fluid intake, postoperative discomfort, or the presence of systemic disorders, e.g., uncontrolled diabetes mellitus, antihypertensive and diuretic medications can precipitate hypovolemia and shock.

This hypovolemia results in a depressed cardiac output, and, in the absence of sufficient increase in peripheral vascular resistance, the vital organs can be damaged: hypotension → impaired tissue perfusion → cellular hypoxia and metabolic damage. However, the redistribution of the blood is a protective mechanism to a certain degree by shunting blood to the vital organs, including the brain, heart, lungs, kidneys and liver. Severe venous pooling of the blood can be seen in the case of a crushing accident, in vasogenic, or septic shock (caused by bacterial exo- or endotoxins of an overwhelming infection), resulting in hypotension, vascular collapse (lowered arterial and venous vascular tone and resistance) due to the insufficient venous return and decreased cardiac output (flow), based on the pressure-equals-flow-times-resistance equation.

Shock may be irreversible if the metabolic damage is resulting in degeneration of cellular organelles, such as "explosion" of mitochondria, autolysosomal activities and disintegration of unit membranes.

The clinical manifestations of shock would include initial restlessness, hyperactivity, anxiety, and rapidly developing stupor, pale, clammy, cold skin, blanched cold mucous membranes and nail beds, tachypnea, hyperpnea, hypotension, tachycardia, weak, thready pulse, anuria, developing metabolic acidosis, cyanosis, decreased muscular tone and mydriasis.

The emergency treatment consists of insurance of an adequate airway and respiration, administration of (10 liter flow) oxygen, if necessary, control of hemorrhage, if present, conservation of body heat, blood transfusions (anticipate if blood loss is more than 15%), plasma volume expanders (saline and lactated Ringer's solution), control of pain, vasopressors, cardiotonics, correction of metabolic acidosis, antibiotics, steroids and monitoring of the vital signs during the observation period. Avoid the unnecessary movement of the patient or premature treatment of wounds or fractures. Keep careful record of corrective and maintenance management, reassure the patient, encourage oral fluid intake. Transfer the patient to the hospital.

Syncope (Fainting, Psychogenic Shock)

This condition is a form of neurogenic shock, a state of temporary, sudden suspension of consciousness related to cerebral ischemia or transient cerebral circulatory insufficiency due to a rapid drop in blood pressure, as seen in peripheral vasodilation with pooling of the blood in the splanchnic and muscular capillaries resulting in reduced cardiac output. This condition may be elicited by various effects on the central nervous system:

a. Fright, fear, anxiety, distressing sights (wound, dental instruments, blood), emotional or psychological stress, pain related vasovagal reactions.

b. Hysteric and anxiety attacks. (In the common hysterical attacks of the emotionally unbalanced patient, falling onto the ground is achieved with impressive gracefulness by avoiding bodily injuries, and no clinical manifestations of common syncope can be revealed.)

c. Stenosis or occlusion of the vertebral arteries, carotids and innominate arteries, as in carotid arch syndrome.

d. Intracranial neoplasm.

The cardiac causes are:

a. Carotid sinus syncope with reflex cardiac inhibition (hypersensitive carotid body baroreceptors react in case of turning the head aside, the pressure of a tight collar, shaving over the carotid sinus, resulting in reflex bradycardia, hypotension, visceral pain, and may be associated with glossopharyngeal neuralgia; also involved is the role of the intercarotid nerve, the branch of the glossopharyngeus, carrying sensory impulses from the carotid sinus to the medulla oblongata).

b. Cardiac diseases, such as cardiac conduction defects, Adams-Stokes syndrome (sudden asystole, extreme hypotension, transient heart block, atrioventricular (A-V) block), paroxysmal ventricular tachycardia, ventricular tachycardia and fibrillation, aortic stenosis or insufficiency, coronary artery disease, myocardial ischemia or infarct.

c. Chronic pulmonary hypertension, embolism and edema (all of these are characterized by the absence of prodromal signs).

The peripheral etiology includes:

a. Postural, or orthostatic, hypotension (during a sudden rise from a recumbent position there is a failure of reflex reaction of the autonomic nervous system at the periphery to prevent a sudden fall in arterial blood pressure as seen in the convalescent stage following prolonged illness with recumbency, diabetic neuropathy, tabes dorsalis, sedatives, antidepressives, antihypertensives).

b. Chronic orthostatic hypotension syndrome which is an extrapyramidal disorder with tremor, ataxia, rigidity, sphincter disturbances due to sympathetic or parasympathetic paralysis, anhydrosis, xerophthalmia, xerostomia, and during micturition as seen in the elderly at night time. Usually, in these cases, the nausea, bradycardia, paleness, and perspiration are absent and the patient regains consciousness rapidly in supine position.

c. Tussive syncope. (If the patient suffers from chronic bronchitis and paroxysms of "explosive" coughing the intrathoracic, intra-abdominal pressure becomes elevated and interferes with the venous return to the heart, diminishes diastolic cardiac filling, and therefore, reduces cardiac output and results in momentary cerebral hypoxia, similar to the Valsalva maneuver or phenomenon in trying to forcefully exhale against a closed glottis.)
Others:

Hyperventilation, severe hemorrhage, or surgical shock, hunger, extreme physical fatigue, poorly ventilated or overheated environment, hypoglycemia, cervical spondylitis, or upper cervical spine congenital anomaly (Klippel-Feil syndrome when the turning of the head results in piercing cervical pain perception, GI distress, nausea, vomiting, vertigo and unconsciousness).

Fleeting faintness may be associated with the milder degree of hypoglycemia, hyperventilation, minor cerebral ischemic attack or a smaller acute internal hemorrhage.

Clinical manifestations: prodromal sensation of giddiness, light-headedness, dizziness, cold perspiration, clammy skin, pallor, nausea, muscle weakness, yawning, tremor, twitching, tachycardia, thready, weak pulse, followed by late manifestations of vomiting, increased micturition urgency, sensation of cold paresthesia, anesthesia of lips, fingers, toes, dyspnea, superficial rapid respiration, onset of sudden profound hypotension, slow, weak pulse, mydriasis and eyes roll up, convulsive movements (due to cerebral hypoxia) and unconsciousness.

If the syncope is prolonged neuron damage can occur at the peripheral areas of the brain.

Emergency treatment of the syncope should extend to correction of the underlying disorder as well as the syncope per se beginning with placing the patient in the Trendelenburg position (except for the pregnant patient who should be rolled on her left side) or lowering the head forward, towards the knees of the sitting patient, eliciting olfactory stimulation by inhalation of vapors of smelling salts, aromatic spirits of ammonia (a Vaporele silk-covered capsule is broken and administered for some minutes), and administration of oxygen at an early stage, if possible. Clear airways by cleaning the mouth and pharynx using suction, loosen tight clothes, apply a cold towel to the head, forehead, face, back of the neck and chest. If blood pressure is low (the systolic lower than the previous diastolic) give phenylephrine (Neo-Synephrine), 1 mg IV, or ephedrine HCl, 25 mg (1 ml) IM, IV, if hypotension persists start saline and lactated Ringer's IV. Record the vital signs and if the pulse rate is less than 60 per minute administer 0.6 mg atropine IV (repeat three times, if necessary). Give emphatic reassurance on recovery, resume dental treatment by gradual repositioning of the patient, perhaps postpone the dental management to the next appointment with oral premedication to prevent syncope.

Syncopal Attacks (Morgagni-Adams-Stokes Syndrome)

This condition is characterized by episodic syncopal attacks due to paroxysmal and transient complete heart block. Trigeminal, glassopharyngeal, vagal stimulation through the afferents from oral, ophthalmic, pharyngeal regions, respiratory, gastrointestinal and genitourinary tracts can elicit increased parasympathetic activity with:

Intermittent or persistent sinoatrial block.
Partial or complete atrioventricular block.
Block of impulse conduction through the bundle of His.
Arrhythmias and tachycardia (tachyarrhythmia).
Fibrillation.
Asystole.

The resulting cerebral ischemia and hypoxia can initiate syncope, convulsions and cardiac standstill (sudden death).

These individuals are most likely over 40 years of age, predominantly suffering from arteriosclerotic heart disease, congenital cardiac disorder, rheumatic heart disease, acute overwhelming fulminant infections, or digitalis intoxication (with bradycardia).

The sudden loss of consciousness is heralded by a fleeting prodromal period with transient dizziness. The longer asystolic period presents paleness, can promote the development of convulsive movements, apnea and mydriasis, the absence of heart sounds, and a marked drop in blood pressure. Persistence of asystole results in cyanosis and possible death.

Syncope may occur at any time or frequency. In general, recovery is rapid with postsyncopal neurologic signs and mental confusion due to the relative cerebral ischemia. Permanent impairment of mental functions are possible.

The emergency medical treatment consists of the Trendelenburg position, application of cold to the face, head and chest, inhalation of aromatic spirits of ammonia, external electric stimulation of the heart in case of cardiac arrest and CPR.

Prevention is extremely important by prophylactic administration of sympathomimetics or atropine.

Since the patient can be maintained on an idioventricular pacemaker discharge it is essential to rule out the existence of a malfunctioning device (pacemaker); if the heart block is complete and the pacemaker fails to function properly resulting syncope is common.

Patients with pacemakers should be kept away from ultrasonic cleaning devices (scalers, presterilizers), microwave ovens (sterilizers), electric pulp testing devices, electrosurgical equipment, and other high frequency and direct current electric equipment.

Tachycardia-Bradycardia Syndrome

Sinus tachycardia is a regular rhythm at a rate of more then 100 systoles per minute originating in the sinus node—the physiologic pacemaker of the heart. The physiologic sinus tachycardia occurs in infancy, childhood or following emotional excitement, anxiety, physical exercise or stress demanding increased cardiac output. The pulse rate may rise to as high as 160 per minute. Pathologic sinus tachycardia occurs in states of hyperthermia, infections, severe acute hemorrhage, anemia, hypoxia, hypotension, shock, cardiac decompensation, pulmonary embolism, vitamin B complex deficiency, hyperthyroidism, etc. Pharmacologic sinus tachycardia can be caused by administration of caffeine, nicotine, alcohol, amyl nitrite and parasympatholytics, sympathomimetics, thyroid hormones, etc.

It is noted that, in normal patients, the pulse rate may increase near the end of the deep inspiration and decrease near the end of the expiration. This condition should not be mistaken for cardiac arrhythmias due to abnormal automacity of cells that reach spontaneously the threshold potential (occurring in the sinus node, in the wall of the atria, in the atrioventricular node, or in the Hiss-Purkinje fibers), abnormalities in conduction, or both.

Sinus bradycardia is a regular rhythmic rate of less than 50 systole per minute. Physiologic sinus bradycardia is usually present during deep sleep and in athletes. Pathologic sinus bradycardia may be seen in carotid sinus sensitivity, ocular hypertension, gagging and vomiting, producing vagal stimulation, acute myocardial infarction, hypothyroidism, etc. Pharmacologic sinus bradycardia may result from digitalis alkaloids, β-adrenergic blockers (e.g., propranolol), Rauwolfia alkaloids (reserpine), central nervous system depressants (morphine). It may also be the part of emotional depression related parasympathomimetic reaction.

Paroxysmal tachycardia is caused most likely by an ectopic physiologic pacemaker or circus cycle located in the myocardium releasing a rapid, rhythmic, regular rate which ends abruptly and recurs at varying frequency. Predisposing factors are organic heart disease, malnutrition and gastrointestinal or autonomic nervous system disturbances, emotional instability, and precipitating factors such as alcohol, tobacco, coffee, menstrual period, exhausting physical stress, infections, allergic reactions, and drug effects like digitalis intoxication. Adult men are most often affected. Manifestations are typical, including sudden onset of sensation of palpitation in the throat or thoracic area, persisting flutter, intense weakness, dyspnea or apnea, faintness and syncope. The attack may last for hours, and the termination of paroxysmal tachycardia is abrupt.

Other causes of tachycardia may include: angina pectoris, hyperthyroidism, leukemia, anemia, pneumonia, cor pulmonale, acute myocardial infarction, infections and inflammations, hyperthermia, aneurysm of the abdominal aorta, etc.

The patient management in sinus tachycardia should be directed towards removal of the underlying pathological condition; the sinus tachycardia itself does not require treatment. Sinus bradycardia resulting in syncope should receive emergency treatment, including the Trendelenburg position, atropine, ephedrine, etc. Prevention of development of syncope in sinus bradycardia should be emphasized indicating graded physical exercise. Paroxysmal tachycardia may be terminated by parasympathetic stimulation, applying pressure on the carotid sinuses (under no circumstances should both carotid sinuses be compressed simultaneously, but alternately for 10 seconds each) or eyeballs to increase vagal tone, eliciting gagging to stimulate glossopharyngeal activity, or administration of various drugs, i.e., Tensilon, to restore the normal rhythm. If organic heart disease is present digitalis should be considered with caution.

Thermal Burns

Burn of the intraoral mucous membranes, the skin of the perioral areas, face, scalp or other areas may occur in a dental office caused by flamed instruments, hot materials, sterilization procedures, electrosurgery or ultraviolet light, etc., producing local lesions of various degrees: first degree burn elicits severe hyperemia. The development of vesicles and involvement of the deeper mucosal areas with retained potential possibility for epithelial regeneration from the appendages (sebaceous and sweat glands, hair follicles) is seen in second degree; the third degree is characterized by deep destruction of tissues which may affect the bone. Large area involvement is not only quite disfiguring but can be life-threatening.

Signs and symptoms include: pain of various intensity, loss of blood plasma and hemoconcentration, blood flow impairment, destruction of erythrocytes (due to local direct heat effect and increase of cell fragility), anemia, hemorrhage, decreased hemoglobin synthesis, syncope and shock. In shock paleness, cold, clammy skin, shallow respiration and weak pulse may be observed, leading to decreased blood supply to the vital organs (brain, liver, kidneys) due to loss of plasma, hemoconcentration, increased blood viscosity and decreased cardiac output.

The treatment of minor burns involves:

Cleaning the area of contamination, removal of foreign materials.

Applying sterile towel in ice water to the hyperemic zone, including the vesicular surface, for about one hour (never allowing the towel to warm up).

Preventing the development of infection.

Protecting the area of burn from further trauma and hindering the adhesion of the cover dressing by using sterile dressing, e.g., Sulfamylon or sulfadiazine.

Minimizing the mobility of the injured area.

Alleviating the pain. Change the dressing and bandage 3 to 4 times a day.

The first degree burn should heal in four days, the second in four weeks, leaving little or no scar; the third degree small lesion leaves scarring and severe contractures, the large lesion is usually treated by skin graft.

Thyroid Crisis (Storm)

A state of active severe hyperthyroidism due to massive release of thyroid hormones into the blood circulation. It occurs most commonly following thyroidectomy (e.g., toxic adenoma with poor preoperative preparation), iodine overdosage, intercurrent severe illness, infections or trauma.

Clinical manifestations of the storm are the following: acute onset of tachycardia, tachyarrhythmia, hyperthermia, restlessness, agitation, diarrhea, mental confusion, fear, expression of impending death, profuse generalized perspiration, flushing and subsequent delirium, peripheral vascular collapse, pulmonary edema, heart failure, unconsciousness and coma.

The treatment includes administration of oxygen, amelioration of the hyperpyrexia by rubbing alcohol, blocking the thyroid hyperactivity:

Propranolol to counteract the β-adrenergic stimulation.

50 to 100 mg IM hydrocortisone.

Norepinephrine to support blood circulation.

Antithyroid medication (methimazole or propylthiouracil; potassium iodide.

Transient Cerebral Ischemic Attacks (TIA) and Cerebrovascular Accident (Stroke) (CVA)

The transient cerebral ischemic attack is a condition indicating the potential danger of cerebral infarction. It is a neurologic disturbance caused by temporary, reversible decrease in blood flow in the distribution of a cerebral artery (such as the internal carotid, anterior cerebral, middle cerebral, or posterior cerebral artery resulting in a deficit in local cerebral function.

The TIA may be caused by arteriosclerotic narrowing of the cerebral arteries, but many times there is a transient change in the brain hemodynamics related to hypotension, hypertension, hypoglycemia, cardiac arrhythmia, minute emboli, smoking, anemia or polycythemia, but in some cases no cause of the temporary attack can be established. The TIA is usually a brief episode, lasting from a few seconds to a few minutes, uncommonly to a few hours. The onset of a CVA is unpredictable and may follow any episode of TIA.

The clinical manifestations of TIA, the signs and symptoms of focal neurologic disturbances, vary, depending on the area of brain affected by the ischemia. Insufficiency of blood circulation occurs in the following blood vessels:

a. Internal carotid artery.

Transient retinal ischemia.

Homolateral reduced visual acuity.

Contralateral weakness, and numbness of the face, arm or leg.

b. Vertebral and Basilar arteries (vertebrobasilar).

Tinnitus.

Dizziness.

Vertigo.

Deafness.

Nystagmus, or disconjugate eye movements, diplopia.

Dysarthria, dysphonia.

Dysphagia.

Deviation of the tongue, soft palate.

Weakness of facial muscles.

Ataxia.

Unilateral or bilateral paresthesia, or anesthesia of the face, arm(s), leg(s).

Impairment of consciousness and convulsions are uncommon.

c. Posterior cerebral artery.

Impairment of visual acuity.

Visual field defect, or transient hemianopia.

Blurred vision.

The insufficient blood supply through the above mentioned arteries can culminate in the ischemia of the entire cerebral hemisphere, resulting in:

Blurred, dim vision.

Slurred, thick speech, dysphasia.

Numbness of one side of the body, contralateral hemiparesis.

Dizziness.

Disturbed thinking.

When TIA precedes a cerebrovascular accident the process is usually related to atherosclerotic thrombosis; it may follow embolism, interrupted cerebral circulation, hypertensive vascular disease, cerebral aneurysm and intracerebral hemorrhage.

The management of TIA depends upon the severity of the attack and is mainly supportive and palliative. It includes giving the patient oxygen to inhale, an ice bag or cold, wet towel on the frontal, occipital regions, making the patient comfortable, giving reassurance, lowering the head and shoulders slightly, loosening restrictive clothing, and preventing injuries if convulsions occur. The emergency measures given in case of stroke are essentially the same as above; in addition, maintaining an open airway in case of unconsciousness; sedatives, narcotics or stimulants are contraindicated. Record vital signs regularly and transport the patient to the hospital emergency room.

Tricuspid Valvular Stenosis and Sudden Death

This condition may be congenital or most commonly caused by development of rheumatic heart disease. There is a decreased right ventricular diastolic filling, lowered cardiac output, elevated venous pressure resulting in clinical manifestations such as fluttering, distress over the great neck veins, fatigue, hepatomegaly due to liver congestion, abdominal distension, pulsating liver, organic heart murmur and possible development of cardiac decompensation.

The patient is usually maintained on digitalis, low sodium intake and restricted physical activity. Severe abdominal distension may require paracentesis of the abdominal wall. (Dental preventive considerations include antibiotic chemoprophylaxis, avoidance of drug interactions and hospital dentistry.)

Urticaria (Hives)

Generalized allergic skin reaction may occur rapidly after administration of the allergen (drug) and may progress quickly into an anaphylactic reaction affecting the respiratory and cardiovascular systems. The most general clinical manifestations are severe pruritus, extreme discomfort, followed by wheals of transient nature that may occur in crops. The severe reaction begins soon after administration of allergen and progresses rapidly into serious, often life-threatening complications. The mild case is treated by antihistamines.

The severe reaction, i.e., anaphylaxis, requires emergency treatment with epinephrine, fluids, cardiovascular drugs and antihistamines.

Venous Air Embolism and Sudden Death

Rapid intravenous injection of 5 to 7 ml of air can be fatal. This lethal air dose may reach the right ventricle, obturate the pulmonary semilunar valve area, enter the pulmonary artery and obliterate its lumen, obstruct pulmonary arterioles and capillaries and interfere with pulmonary blood circulation, creating pulmonary, cardiac and cerebral hypoxemia, pulmonary hypertension and edema, reflex systemic hypotension and bradycardia, diminished cardiac output, dyspnea, cyanosis, shock, coma; in some cases sudden death is witnessed. The auscultation may reveal murmur over the right ventricle, indicating the presence of air in the heart chamber.

The emergency treatment begins with CPR. The patient is quickly transferred to the hospital emergency ward.

chapter

5

Specific Infections the Dentist May Encounter

LEVENTE Z. BODAK-GYOVAI

Viral Hepatitis

Etiology

Hepatitis A virus (HAV); hepatitis B virus (HBV); non-A, non-B type.

Diagnostic Considerations

Since the dentist will always meet undiagnosed infectious individuals, the main infectious hazard to the dentist is the patient who is not known to be infective for viral hepatitis. To screen all the patients for seropositivity before dental treatment is not practical. To exercise the recommended protective measures (gloves, etc.) when practicing dentistry will not provide absolute protection against viral hepatitis since ample opportunity exists to break these protective barriers (puncture of the gloves, etc.).

The essential point is to screen a subpopulation of high risk patients, to identify their infectivity and to take precautionary measures when indicated. Screening consists of a health questionnaire and complete medical history with concentrated attention on past exposure to or infection with viral hepatitis in high risk patients. The history should include the following data.

Past history of having had hepatitis (jaundice, liver disease, dark urine).

Had positive HB$_s$AG by radioimmunoassay (RIA).

Presented clinical manifestations of hepatitis (will be described later).

Members of the health profession, including clinical and laboratory staff.

Professional and volunteer blood donors.

Excluded as blood donor in the past.

Received several transfusions or blood products.

Received prophylactic or therapeutic injections for any reasons.

Cancer patients, victims of leukemia, leprosy, mongolism.

Chronic hemodialysis patients, chronic renal failure states.

Renal transplant individuals.

Patients treated in mental institutions.

Drug addicts.

Tattooed.

Prisoners.

Woman in childbearing age.

Experienced acupuncture.

Immigrants from the tropical countries, in general.

Military personnel.

Sometimes the history of special medical management of an individual can indicate a high risk viral hepatitis patient (who has received fresh pooled hyperimmune gamma globulin serum, corticosteroids and sedatives and is confined to limited physical activity, along with a special diet).

It must be noted that negative or positive past histories of hepatitis did not correlate well with antigen carrier states.

The spectrum of clinical disorders of viral hepatitis ranges from transient anicteric infection to fulminant fatal liver necrosis. Subclinical or clinical manifestations of anicteric or icteric hepatitis are similar. The preicteric phase (incubation period or prodromal stage) is characterized by early tiredness, chills, fever, weakness, malaise, cephalgia, sore throat, dysgeusia, anorexia, abdominalgia, diarrhea, myalgia, painful migratory arthritis, urticaria, erythema, maculopapular rash and dark urine in the late phase. The icteric phase involves jaundice (or anicteric), generalized pruritus, nausea, vomitus, abdominal distension, anemia and purpuric manifestations.

HAV is not known to be related to carrier states. The patient is infective two weeks before and about two weeks after the onset of the icteric phase. The preicteric phase is 15 to 90 days.

HBV is known to be associated with carrier states—asymptomatic carrier states may follow both subclinical and clinical HBV infections. The patient is potentially infective during HB antigenemia, including patients who are in the incubation period as well as those who are asymptomatic carriers (apparently normal, healthy individuals). Table 5.1 shows the results of serologic tests.

Non-A, non-B type may well be associated with carrier states and chronic liver disease. Although this disease appears to be common, not much is known about it, no laboratory tests are available to identify the causative agent or antigens.

At this point it is necessary to emphasize the need for protective measures of dentist and staff during any contact with saliva and blood contamination from the oral cavity of the patient—the basic milieu of dental activities—and to prevent the transmission of the infective agents to patients.

Dentists working in a high-volume practice have ample opportunity to encounter HBV carriers. For this reason they should regard all of their patients as infectious with hepatitis, unless proven otherwise. The environment to practice dentistry is special, involving sharp instruments, jagged teeth confined in a crowded, small area and contaminated by blood stained saliva.

The dentist and staff should follow routine protective measures in treating known or suspected infectious hepatitis patients, HBV positive chronic carriers, individuals presenting active infectious hepatitis and those who have a positive history of hepatitis, but refuse an RIA test (RIA negatives should be retested for two consecutive times at three-month intervals).

1. Personnel. The providers of care should wear protective surgical clothing: mask, surgical gloves (vinyl), glasses

Table 5.1
Serologic Tests and What They Indicate

	Acute B Hepatitis	Carrier State
HB$_s$Ag	The marker of viremia appears as early as 6 days after exposure and gradually disappears during convalescence (Radioimmunoassay is false negative in 2%).	The indicator of carrier state, appears on viremia and persists, probably for life.
Anti-HB$_s$ (HB$_s$-Ab)	Appears a few weeks after the HB$_s$Ag is no longer positive and may persist for years.	Fails to appear in carriers.
HB$_e$Ag (Core Ag represents DNA polymerase associated with HB$_s$AG)	Indicator of active HBV reduplication and appears on viremia, disappears during recovery	Indicates infectivity, appears on viremia and persists for many years.
Anti-HB$_e$ (HB$_e$-Ab)	Persists for many years, if present.	
Anti-HB$_c$ (HB$_c$-Ab)	Indicator of active reduplication of HBV, appears soon after HB$_s$Ag positivity, (the titer is over 1:50), and declines in later years.	Appears following HB$_s$ Ag positivity and persists for years as a marker of past HBV infection. Consistently present in carriers indicating high infectivity.

(should be routine for all dental procedure), headdress, gown and pants (scrub suit), and shoe covers (overshoes). These are to be collected in linen hampers before leaving the operating area and followed by proper laundry procedures.

Minor shaving cuts and abrasions are to be covered by waterproof tape.

Avoid the use of spray and aerosol products to prevent contamination of the conjunctivae or the respiratory tract (inhalation).

In case of an accidental puncture wound with contaminated material, IM hepatitis B hyperimmune gamma globulin serum should be given for passive immunization within hours of the injury and repeated four weeks later.

Hand washing is essential (with or without the gloves) with warm water and soap to remove saliva and blood; the hands should then be thoroughly disinfected (described later).

Eating, drinking and smoking are not permitted in the operating area.

The telephone, door knob, camera, equipment, pen, pencil and paper work (chart) cannot be handled with contaminated hands. If it is necessary to touch these, use paper towels and disinfect them. The soiled paper must be incinerated.

2. The operating area and equipment should be suitable for isolation and maintenance: a closed area, laminated air flow, Phenol Gard mat at the door, plumbing system with back flow traps, independent (portable) suction unit, disposable drapes for the dental chair and stool. The service personnel should follow the same precautionary steps.

3. A substerile area should be used to store and handle supplies and to pass instruments and materials (one way process) to the sterile area.

4. A sterilizing area should be maintained to clean and sterilize contaminated instruments.

5. Dental supplies and consumable materials should be handled during treatment procedures as contaminated and should be properly disposed of (see below). All impressions, models, prosthetic devices, etc., are to be wrapped in bleach soaked paper towels prior to forwarding to the laboratory.

6. Instruments. Use disposable instruments (needles, local anesthetic cartridges, etc.), if possible, and dispose of them by using a double plastic bag technique for incineration.

Nondisposable instruments, after being thoroughly scrubbed and washed (wear heavy duty rubber gloves), are to be sterilized (complete destruction of all microorganisms) by autoclaving (120°C, 8 kg, for 15 minutes) or by exposure to dry heat 160°C for 60 minutes).

The instruments may be stored prior to sterilization in a disinfectant (3% aqueous solution of concentrate phenolic detergent, or Cidex—2% glutaraldehyde).

7. The equipment, operating area walls, floors and rubber goods should be disinfected (chemical reduction of pathogenic microorganisms, except spores) using Phenol Gard/bleach (mix 3 ml in 0.5 liter of water). Any contaminated (blood stained, saliva spotted) dental area or equipment should be covered with a tissue soaked in phenolic solution for 30 minutes and subsequently washed with soap and water.

The portable suction bottle should be rinsed with Phenol Gard/bleach.

Provided the protective measurements are taken, only the emergency type of dental treatment (oral condition related to the short-term effect on the patient's function, pain or esthetics) can be performed on a patient having active viral hepatitis.

It should be remembered that, if the patient presents a questionable history of hepatitis (see the high risk category), unless the serologic tests can be carried out, the patient must be managed as an infective carrier during dental treatment. The serology should include the HB_sAg, or at best, the anti-HB_c.

Comprehensive routine dental treatment (oral condition related to the long-term effect on the patient, e.g., crowns, bridges, orthodontics) is allowed upon complete recovery from viral hepatitis, if all the serologic tests indicate no infectivity, including the absence of abnormal bleeding and normal liver test results, a state which may be reached in the six-month postinfective period. At any rate the patient's physician should be consulted on this vital issue.

Tuberculosis

Etiology

Mycobacterium tuberculosis.

Diagnostic Characteristics

Asymptomatic primary infection occurs in 99% of individuals without clinical tuberculosis, resulting in tuberculin hypersensitivity. In this setting, pulmonary tuberculosis and/or extrapulmonary tuberculosis may develop later.

Chronic pulmonary tuberculosis may be suspected, presenting insidious onset of fatigue, weight loss, anorexia, chilliness, afternoon fever, night sweats, hoarseness, cough, dyspnea, chest pain, sputum production, hemoptysis, dysphagia, pharyngeal ulcers, otitis media and anal pain.

The chest roentgenogram may indicate changes suggestive of tuberculosis, and the sputum smear may be positive for acid fast bacteria.

Extrapulmonary tuberculosis may involve any tissue in the body, producing painful oral ulcers, tuberculous gingivitis, sialadenitis, postextraction nonhealing complications with "cold abscess" and tuberculous osteomyelitis, pharyngeal ulcers, tuberculous laryngitis, cervical lymphadenitis (scrofula), esophageal and stomach ulcers, bleeding duodenal ulcer, tuberculous enteritis with hemorrhage, joint stiffness and swelling, bone pain on motion and gait and paralysis.

Miliary tuberculosis and tuberculous meningitis are grave generalized consequences.

General Management

The drugs of choice include isoniazid, rifampin, streptomycin, ethambutol and paraaminosalicylic acid, in various combinations.
(Preventive BCG vaccination decreases the incidence of clinical illness and induces tuberculin positivity, but is of no use in a tuberculin positive person.)

Dental Considerations

The dentist may contract an infection from the oral cavity of the patient suffering from pulmonary tuberculosis; for this reason the dentist should have PPD (tuberculin test) at yearly intervals. The negative PPD in a nonfebrile and relatively well individual is strong evidence against tuberculosis. The good medical Hx is essential to rule out special risk factors related to tuberculosis:

Was the patient hospitalized for tuberculosis?

Did the patient receive treatment for tuberculosis?

Has he lived with a tuberculous patient?

Has the patient had long-standing PPD positivity?

If the patient is not taking medications, were antituberculous medications prescribed?

Has the patient undergone PPD conversion (negative converted to positive)?

Has the patient received corticosteroids?

Are there predisposing factors present to develop poor resistance, such as malnutrition, excessive ozone exposure (sun lamp), unusual physical exertion, psychological stress, chronic debilitating diseases; occupational risks of polluted air such as are encountered by miners, tunnelers, quarrymen, asbestos workers?

Suspected patients with tuberculosis should be referred to a physician prior to dental treatment for a chest roentgenograph, sputum culture and thorough physical examination.

Patients presenting a positive history of tuberculosis who are PPD positive, or who undergo conversion from negative to positive PPD, must receive a chest x-ray examination and other studies to determine the presence or absence of active pulmonary tuberculosis.

If the patient does not take the prescribed antituberculous medications, he should be considered infectious.

Skin test converters (rule out BCG) without active disease should be offered INH prophylaxis. Patients with active tuberculosis should allow at least 6 months to elapse on effective antituberculous therapy prior to elective dental treatment.

The dentist and auxiliary personnel must take special personal protective measures (mask, gloves, etc.) and special precautions relative to instrument sterilization if treating patients with active or suspected pulmonary tuberculosis, or potentially infective extrapulmonary tuberculous patients with open and draining wounds.

Syphilis

Etiology

Treponema pallidum.

Diagnostic Characteristics

The *early syphilis* (less than four years' duration) presents:

1. An incubation period of two to six weeks.

2. Initial (primary) lesions (chancres) as painless, solitary, circumscribed lesions accompanied by painless, freely movable, hard, regional lymphadenopathy. The chancre heals in a few weeks, the lymphadenopathy resolves in a few months.

3. Secondary manifestations may be seen in six to eight weeks of infection as firm, freely movable, painless, generalized, superficial lymphadenitis, a reddish, macular, mucocutaneous rash lasting for one to two months, associated with or followed by reddish papules lasting two to four weeks. Relapses and exacerbations of mucocutaneous manifestations (condyloma latum, split papules, perioral circinate and other varieties of papules, patchy loss of hair, mucous patches (occur in about one-third of those infected), ulceromembranous pharyngitis, tonsillitis causing hoarseness); "meningeal rash" resulting in headaches, nocturnal ostealgia with periostitis, and ophthalmic involvement are common. This condition terminates in *early latent* (asymptomatic) syphilis of less than two years and *late latent* stage of greater than two years. The individual is infectious during the incubation period and the early stage up to the latent stage.

Late (tertiary) syphilis (more than four years' postinfection duration) presents:

1. Late latent (asymptomatic) syphilis (dormant).

2. Late symptomatic syphilis: destructive skin lesions, gumma involving any part of the body such as palate and nose (rhinopharyngitis mutilans), neurolues as central nervous system involvement with cranial nerve disorders, tabes dorsalis, general paresis and cardiovascular syphilis as aneurysm of the aorta.

Congenital (prenatal) syphilis presents:

1. Early congenital syphilis (occurs in children less than two years old) manifested by visceral involvement, osteochondritis, nasopharyngeal discharge, cutaneous rash.

2. Late congenital syphilis (manifested in the older children) presents rhagades, frontal bossing, knee joint and tibial changes, saddle nose, Hutchinson's triad, paresis and tabes.

Laboratory Diagnosis

Serologic tests (e.g., rapid plasma reagin) may be reactive four weeks after the infection, including congenital syphilis (as early as twenty weeks fetal life) and seropositivity is often maintained for a post-treatment surveillance period. In about 10% the "false" seroreactivity (malnutrition, heroin addiction, lupus, malaria) requires additional specific treponemal tests. Treponemal antibody tests (FTA = fluorescent treponemal antibody test/TPI = treponema immobilization test) are essential to rule out "false" positive seroreactivity.

General Management

Adequate parenteral antibiotic (penicillin) therapy—the "gunshot" treatment—is practiced as accepted by schedules. The patient is noninfective 2 to 5 days after the initiation of adequate treatment. Decline of seroreactivity is expected within a few months in case of early syphilis. Serorelapse (back to positive) presenting infective mucocutaneous lesions may be due to inadequate treatment or reinfection on new exposure. Serologic nonreactivity may be reached within a few years during the course of untreated late syphilis (the FTA/TPI may remain reactive for the length of the life). The treatment of early congenital syphilis is usually massive, the late congenital syphilis (malformations) requires special syphilologic consultations and laboratory evaluations.

Dental Considerations

Syphilis may be contracted as an occupational disease during the professional duties of the dentist and staff through the disrupted continuity of the integument as well as the conjunctivae and oral mucosa, since bacteremia is common in active syphilis, manifesting peripheral lesions, and the oral cavity is one of the major sources of dissemination of infection by *T. pallidum*.

In case of an accidental exposure to infection the scheduled prophylactic treatment and follow-up serologic tests should commence.

If emergency dental treatment is necessary in an infective individual, the dentist should wear a mask, spectacles, surgical gloves, avoid aerosol and droplet generation (high speed drills, ultrasonic scaler, compressed air), and exercise scrupulous disinfection and sterilization procedures.

The complete health history should elicit much information about the disease, methods and adequacy of treatment and the recurrence of clinical manifestations. No special precautions are required for patients who were adequately treated for syphilis.

Gonococcal Infection

Etiology

Neisseria gonorrhoeae.

Diagnostic Characteristics

Symptoms include abdominal pain, urethritis, dysuria, urgency, frequency, mucoid discharge, temperature above 38°C, prostration, migratory polyarthritis or solitary pyogenic arthritis. Intermittent gonococcemia may present recurrent fever, septic joints and skin rash. Genital or oral mucous membrane invasion (a favorite location for gonococcal infection) is common, causing purulent inflammatory reaction. More than 30% of cases are complicated by extragenital involvement via hematologic dissemination, including rheumatism, meningitis and endocarditis. The definite diagnosis can be established by isolation of gonococci from the infected area. There is no blood test available to detect gonorrhea.

General Management

Treatment consists of penicillin or tetracycline. The disease may persist for decades if untreated.

Dental Considerations

Active gonorrhea is a lingering threat to the dentist providing dental treatment to the infective patient. Oral mucosal lesions are secondary to infected genital lesions (either direct or by the hands), or related to the metastatic spread of gonococcal infection: swollen, inflamed gingivae, similar to acute necrotizing ulcerative gingivitis, whitish-yellow adherent mucous patches with sloughing, leaving bright areas with numerous hemorrhagic points involving any part of the oral mucosa such as the soft palate, tongue, buccal mucosa, as well as asymptomatic tonsillitis, pharyngitis. Gonococcus may infect the conjunctivae of the dentist. When the patient presents a positive history of venereal disease, questions should be directed to determine which form of VD was diagnosed, was adequate treatment completed, were post-treatment evaluation and follow-up care performed, did the clinical manifestations return. Positive responses indicate referral to the physician for medical evaluation prior to elective dental treatment.

chapter
6

Nutritional Evaluation of the Dental Patient

LEVENTE Z. BODAK-GYOVAI

Although the classic signs and symptoms of major nutritional disorders are seldom established, the subclinical or borderline clinical manifestations of nutritional deficiency diseases are not uncommon.

The prevention oriented dental profession recognizes the role of nutrition in clinical practice and applies nutritional principles to oral health. It requires the cooperative efforts of patients, dentist and often a professional individual (nutritional biochemist, dietetic intern) to assess the dietary aspects of the patient.

A patient's nutritional state is determined by qualitative and quantitative dietary characteristics, food intake (a cardinal component), absorption, utilization, storage and elimination of food substances. The individual levels of caloric requirement depend on age, sex, body size, basal metabolic rate, physical activity, environmental temperature and the presence of systemic disease. For example, nutritional deficiency may be related to the state of increased general metabolic requirements, high fever, nutritional demands of hyperthyroidism, hyperactivity, massive chemotherapeutic intake, extreme cold or hot environment, heavy physical work, a high level of carbohydrate consumption, and the dietary restrictions of hypothyroid and obese patients. The development and continuous turn-over of soft and hard tissues and the repair and replacement of injured tissues are intimately dependent on nutrition.

In relation to oral health, nutritional factors play a clear role in both caries and wound healing, the maintenance of integrity of mucous membranes and the development of periodontal disease. A sensitive indicator and most common symptom of nutritional deficiency is the soreness of the mucosal lining of the oral cavity, including the tongue surfaces.

Subsets of population which have been shown to be at increased nutritional risk are: the poor of any age, the geriatric age group, especially if living alone, and individuals eating erratically or consuming monotonous or restricted diets which limit the variety and/or amount of food eaten.

Obesity is widespread with a higher prevalence in females than in males and in lower than higher socioeconomic levels. Visual inspection will usually identify the obese patient. More specific determination is allowed by the use of the ponderal index and weight-height reference tables. Risk patients can be easily identified by asking a simple question: "Do you follow any special dietary restriction?"

The same question may lead to information on medical problems which require therapeutic modification of the diet and frequency of meals. These include diabetes mellitus, hypertension, gout, hyperlipoproteinemias, chronic renal disease, gastrointestinal disorders and food allergy. Other problems of nutritional significance which may be revealed in the medical history include malabsorption syndromes, alcoholism, cholecystopathies and hepatic diseases. Normal physiologic states which increase nutrient needs, such as puberty,

158

Table 6.1
Signs and Symptoms of Nutrient Deficiencies

Tissue	Abnormality	Nutrient(s)/Disorder
Oral mucosa	Scrotal tongue, gingival hyperplasia, marginal and generalized gingivitis, periodontal disease, keratinizing metaplasia	A hypovitaminosis
	Hyperpigmentation	E hypovitaminosis
	Gingival hemorrhages, ecchymoses, postoperative purpura	K hypovitaminosis
	Marginal gingivitis, gingival spongy swellings (present in edentulous patient too), dark red hyperemia, hyperplasia, hypertrophy, hemorrhages, ulceration and necrosis, severe periodontal disease	C hypovitaminosis
	Bleeding (due to thrombocytopenia), infection (related to leukopenia), fiery red, sore-smooth glossitis	B_{12} and folacin hypovitaminosis
	Glossodynia, stomatitis, bright red inflamed oral mucosa, beefy red, swollen, scarlet glossitis with papillary atrophy, crenation, fissuration, marginal and generalized gingivitis	Niacin hypovitaminosis
	Stomatitis, burning and soreness of oral mucosa, marginal and generalized gingivitis, angular stomatitis, cheilosis, magenta tongue: purplish, red, fissured glossitis with ultimate central atrophy of filiform and fungiform papillae (there is an early hypertrophy of filiforms)	Ariboflavinosis (B_2)
	Hypertrophy of the filiform and fungiform lingual papillae	Thiamin (B_1) deficiency
	Stomatitis	Pyridoxine (B_6) deficiency
	Pallor of mucous membranes, glossodynia, atrophy of lingual papillae	Iron deficiency
	Enlarged thyroid; in myxedema the tongue is large, edematous, frequently interfering with speech (due to interstitial accumulation of water and myxedema protein)	Iodine deficiency
	Xerostomia, bright red glossitis with atrophy of papillae, crenation	Protein deficiency (kwashiorkor)
	Firm, yellowish, waxy nodules, verrucous, keratotic plaques	Lipid proteinosis
	Macroglossia, gingival hyperplasia	Mucopolysaccharidosis (Hurler's Syndrome)
		Lipid metabolism
	Periodontal disease, poor postoperative healing, dysgeusia	*A.* Hand-Schülller-Christian disease
	Gingival hyperplasia, severe periodontal disease	*B.* Letterer-Siwe disease
Lips, skin, eyes	Xeroderma (generalized dryness of the skin), follicular hyperkeratosis ("goose flesh" skin), xerosis conjunctivae xerophthalmia (dryness of conjunctivae, corneae), decreased lacrimation, keratomalacia (necrosis and perforation of the cornea, prolapse of the iris, lens disintegration, Bitot's spots ranging from small air vesicles of conjunctivae to small erosions, white coating extending to the limbus of the cornea), nyctalopia, hemeralopia, photophobia and loss of light reflex.	A hypovitaminosis
	Sparse and coarse hair, keratinization of lips	A hypervitaminosis

Table 6.1— *Continued*

Tissue	Abnormality	Nutrient(s)/Disorder
	Cutaneous ecchymoses	K hypovitaminosis
	Subcutaneous ecchymoses, cutaneous hemorrhages, perifollicular and scorbutic petechiae (larger and darker than other forms of purpura, easily induced by tourniquet and appearing mostly on hairy skin areas), hyperkeratotic hair follicles (folliculosis)	C hypovitaminosis
	Hemorrhages and infections, lemon-yellow skin shade, palmar hyperpigmentation	B_{12} and folacin deficiency
	Pellagrous dermatitis (chronic, inelastic, fissured, erythematous, dry areas with hyperkeratinization, desquamation, deep pigmentation), characteristic pattern of skin thickening (Casal's necklace) of sunlight exposed areas, malar and supraorbital pigmentation.	Niacin deficiency
	Circumoral hyperemia, angular cheilosis, chapped lips, shallow ulcers, paleness of lips, cheilosis, scaly, greasy, erythematous, seborrheic dermatitis with moist, weeping, raw-red lesions, dyssebaccia (oiliness, fissuring and exfoliation) especially at nasolabial folds, alae nasi, scrotal and vulval dermatosis, photophobia, diffuse burning, itching conjunctivitis, lacrimation, corneal ulceration, angular palpebritis, corneal vascularization	Ariboflavinosis
	Angular cheilosis	Pyridoxine hypovitaminosis
	Swollen edematous lips, nose, eyelids, suborbital tissues	Iodine deficiency
	Alopecia, dry, desquamating (leaving raw areas), hyperkeratotic, and pigmented dermatosis, angular cheilosis, thin, fine, dry and brittle hair which can be pulled out easily, the dyspigmented hair color changes to lighter (the skin changes are unlimited to areas exposed to sunlight)	Kwashiorkor
	Corneal clouding	Hurler's syndrome
	Pallor, cold skin	Hyperpotassemia
	Firm, yellowish-white waxy skin nodules, verrucous plaques, keratotic papules	Lipid proteinosis
	Exophthalmos	Hand-Schüller-Christian disease
	Exanthems, purpura, erythema and ecchymoses	Letterer-Siwe disease
Teeth, bone	In children: enamel hypoplasia, retarded eruption rate	A hypovitaminosis
	Precocious skeletal development, clubbing of the fingers	A hypervitaminosis
	Rickets and osteomalacia with bone pains, pseudofractures, pathologic fractures, skeletal deformities (due to undermineralization), growth retardation in children with retarded eruption rate, enamel hypoplasia (rachitic teeth), pronounced periosteal thickening Active rickets in children: beading of ribs, painless enlargement of epiphyses, craniotabes Arrested rickets in adolescent: frontal and parietal bossing, bow legs, or knock-knees, thorax deformities Adult osteomalacia: local or general skeletal deformities	D hypovitaminosis

Table 6.1— *Continued*

Tissue	Abnormality	Nutrient(s)/Disorder
	Painful enlargement of epiphyses, bone and joint aches, hemarthroses, subperiosteal hemorrhages, severe mobility of the teeth	C hypovitaminosis
	Enamel hypoplasia of developing dentition	E hypovitaminosis
	Retarded growth and permanent physical stunting	Kwashiorkor
	Negative effects on bone formation and resorption, development and mineralization of dentition	Calcium deficit
	Bone changes	Hypocupremia (copper)
	Resistance to dental caries in case of fluorosis (excess fluoride), mottling of enamel, vague pains in the small joints, increased periosteal bone growth, osteophyte formation	Fluorine
	Intimately associated with calcium metabolism of bones and teeth, e.g., severe rickets and related low phosphorus diet	Phosphorus
	Dwarfed stature, hypertelorism with saddle nose, dental diasthemas	Hurler's syndrome
	Single or multiple "punched out" skeletal lesions	Hand-Schüller-Christian disease
	Diffuse involvement of the skeleton	Letterer-Siwe disease
Central and peripheral nervous system and other effects	Reduced resistance to infection, keratinizing metaplasia of epithelial cells, e.g., salivary gland ducts	A hypovitaminosis
	Irritability, severe headaches, drowsiness, vomiting, hepatosplenomegaly	A hypervitaminosis
	Hypocalcemic tetany, anorexia, muscular hypotonia, muscle weakness, waddling gait	D hypovitaminosis
	Generalized calcinosis (due to hypercalcemia and calcium phosphate deposition in the mucoproteins of the matrix) affecting synovial membranes of joints, kidneys, myocardium, pulmonary alveoli, parathyroid glands, pancreas, skin, arteries, lymph nodes, cornea, conjunctivae and, in general, negative influence on skeletal integrity	D hypervitaminosis
	Depressing effects in CNS, vascular, muscular and hematopoietic systems	E hypovitaminosis
	Purpurae, e.g., epistaxes, CVA, hematuria, GI bleeding	K hypovitaminosis
	Malaise, weakness, lassitude, dyspnea, intramuscular and other hemorrages, pallor, hypotension, syncope and all the manifestations of scurvy, including decreased resistance to infection, poor wound healing	C hypovitaminosis
	Easy fatigability, weakness, tiredness, dyspnea, headaches, orthostatic hypotension with faintness, syncope, palpitations, neurotic and neuropsychiatric problems "megaloblastic madness" (depression, paranoid ideation, irritability, sleeplessness, forgetfulness), neurologic symptoms (symmetrical paresthesias, burning, tingling sensation of extremities, anesthesias, decreased position and vibration sense, diminished tendon reflexes, unsteady gait), hepatosplenomegaly, diarrhea, low grade fever	B_{12} and folacin deficiency

Table 6.1— *Continued*

Tissue	Abnormality	Nutrient(s)/Disorder
	Weakness, lassitude, anxiety, irritability, depression, progressive dementia, disorientation, confusion, delirium, forgetfulness, hallucinations, digestive disturbances, anorexia, severe weight loss, diarrhea, profuse salivation and esophagitis, urethritis, vaginitis, plus all the other signs and symptoms of pellagra	Niacin deficiency
	Multiple neuritis, sensory disturbances, fatigue, foot and wrist drop, motor weakness, loss of ankle jerk, muscle pain, tightness and tenderness, nocturnal muscle cramps, cardiovascular manifestations of beriberi such as progressive congestive cardiac decompensation, cardiomegaly, circulatory insufficiency, violent palpitations, tachycardia, severe dyspnea, generalized edema, intense precordial pain, cyanosis	Thiamin hypovitaminosis
	Mental confusion, depression	Pyridoxine hypovitaminosis
	Psychomotor derangement, low body weight, moon face, apathy, anorexia, marked pitting, muscle weakness, edema of legs, ascites, diarrhea, poor resistance to infection due to severe protein deficiency relative to calories	Kwashiorkor
	Hyperirritability, increased neuromuscular excitability, and muscle contractibility, including myocardial rhythm and typical tetany, decreased blood coagulation	Hypocalcemia
	Metastatic calcifications, muscle rigor, depressed nerve conductivity	Hypercalcemia
	Spinal nerve compression, muscle weakness, paresthesia, paralysis	Fluorosis
	Thyroid enlargement (goiter) related to hypertrophy and hyperplasia	Iodine deficiency
	Plummer-Vinson syndrome, koilonychia	Iron deficiency
	Neuromuscular hyperirritability, athetoid movements, carpopedal spasm, positive Chvostek sign, semicoma	Magnesium deficit
	Narcosis	Magnesium excess
	Weakness, lassitude, apathy, anorexia, peripheral vascular collapse, nausea, hyperexcitability, muscle cramps, convulsions	Sodium and chlorine deficiency
	Muscle weakness, decreased muscular irritability, diminished reflexes, paralysis, mental confusion, paralytic ileus, cardiac and respiratory failure	Hypopotassemia
	Mental confusion, weakness, paresthesia of the extremities, disturbed cardiac rhythm, peripheral vascular collapse	Hyperpotassemia
	Mental retardation, hepatosplenomegaly	Hurler's syndrome
	Diabetes insipidus	Hand-Schüller-Christian disease
	Malaise, irritability, hepatosplenomegaly, lymphadenopathy, diffuse involvement of visceral organs	Letterer-Siwe disease

Table 6.2
Age Related Weight/Height Values

	Male					Female			
Height (cm)[a]	Age (yrs) and Weight (kg)[b]				Height (cm)[a]	Age (yrs) and Weight (kg)[b]			
	5 yrs	10 yrs	15 yrs	25+		5 yrs	10 yrs	15 yrs	25+
96–119	15–22				96–119	15–22			
119–152	22–41				119–152	22–41			
145–188		42–72			142–180		36–63		
	Small frame	Medium frame	Large frame			Small frame	Medium frame	Large frame	
157	52	56	60		147	43	46	50	
160	54	58	62		150	44	47	52	
162	55	59	63		152	45	48	53	
165	56	60	65		154	47	50	54	
167	58	62	67		157	48	51	56	
170	60	63	68		160	49	53	57	
172	61	66	71		162	51	54	58	
175	63	67	72		165	52	56	60	
177	65	69	74		167	53	58	62	
180	67	71	77		170	55	59	64	
182	69	73	79		172	57	61	66	
185	71	75	81		175	59	63	67	
187	73	77	83		177	61	65	70	
190	75	80	85		180	63	67	72	
193	77	82	87		182	65	68	74	

[a] with shoes (about 2.5 cm heels).
[b] in regular indoor clothing.
Composed by the author based on measurements at Diagnostic Clinic, University of Pennsylvania School of Dental Medicine; data exhibited by both the Baldwin-Wood and Metropolitan Life Insurance Companies.

pregnancy and lactation, should also alert the clinician to the possibility of nutritional inadequacy.

When a high risk malnutrition patient is identified by the above described criteria, or for any other pathologic reason, including oral clinical manifestations (rampant caries, periodontal disease, ulcerations), or the diet is of questionable adequacy or frankly inadequate, nutritional counseling should be included in the dental treatment plan.

Clinical Manifestations Related to Dietary Abnormalities

The clinical manifestations of nutritional deficiencies are not absolutely diagnostic by themselves; however, these abnormalities may indicate a need for further investigation. The oral cavity is one of the first sites where signs and symptoms of nutrient deficiency appear. The clinician must be alert to detect subtle changes in oral tissues which are suggestive of poor nutritional status.

Table 6.1 summarizes signs and symptoms of several common nutrient deficiencies.

It is generally accepted that a 22-year-old, healthy person—for example, a 70-kg male or a 50-kg female—living in a 20°C environment maintaining minor physical activity, consumes 240 and 120 kcal[1] per

---

[1] Protein is consumed at about 4 calories per gram; carbohydrate at about 4 calories per gram; fat at about 9 calories per gram.

hour, respectively. When caloric and protein intake are limited to about the same degree, the condition of marasmus may develop. The child is "skin and bones." Severe caloric deficiency in adults may result in cachexia. A self-imposed severe weight loss due to excessive fasting, self-induced vomiting, abuse of purgatives, promotion of noncarbohydrate diet, or excessively heavy physical exercise may cause anorexia nervosa, characterized by progressive malnutrition, depression, unhappiness, irritability and often agitation.

Severe undernutrition is characterized by low weight, mental and physical depression, lethargy, diminished skin folds, exaggerated skeletal prominences and decreased elasticity of the integument.

Obesity may be indicated by increased body weight in relation to height and size of the skeleton (Table 6.2). Excessive subcutaneous adiposity may advance by age as measured by the thickness of the skin folds. The upper adult limits are:

	Male	Female
Triceps	2 cm	3 cm
Subscapular	2 cm	3 cm
Abdominal girth	3 cm	4 cm

Since a muscular individual may be overweight without being obese, direct practical indices are preferred:

a. Ponderal index $= \dfrac{\text{height}}{\sqrt[3]{\text{weight}}}$

b. Body mass index $= \dfrac{\text{weight}}{\text{height}^2} \times 100$

Anxiety As Related to the Dental Patient

HERMAN SEGAL

Patients frequently report for emergency dental treatment to private offices with the idea that they have an "ordeal" awaiting them. This "ordeal" can be subdivided into several categories. The foremost is the fear of impending pain both from the problem that exists and pain that might be induced from the tests taken and the therapeutic procedures which will follow to treat the problem. These fears and trepidations help promote a state of apprehension and anxiety in some. The patient and, at times, the practitioner are not aware that the process is developing. The patient may state he is "nervous" and "just doesn't like going to the dentist." The dentist who may have heard these and other similar statements develops a "thick hide." This occurs as a protective mechanism and serves as a defense on the dentist's part. Very simply, if this type patient is asked, "How can we make treatment more acceptable?" or "How can I help you relax?" the patient often responds in a direct manner. Depending on his educational background and past dental experiences, he may be surprised that someone cares enough to ask. A very simple response may be put forth such as "Is there any way that I can avoid getting a needle? It's not the needle but my heart seems to pound afterward." This is a common response. Future behavior can be modified by informing the patient that there are anesthetics that can be used that will not cause this pain. This should be stated in language the patient will understand. Most patients are not familiar with the phar-macological actions of epinephrine. This and all questions should be answered in language that is comprehended by the patient. The patient's "complaint" is only one of many messages that are unspoken and therefore unreceived in the dentist-patient encounter.

It is logical to assume that if more messages are relayed and thereby received, a better overall rapport will develop in the doctor/patient relationship.

I. Anxiety

In order to manage a patient's anxiety, it is vital to first define the process known as anxiety, and then to establish the diagnostic criteria.

According to Webster's dictionary, anxiety is (1) a condition of mental uneasiness or worry about the future; concern about what may happen; (2) a highly emotional state characterized by exaggerated or unfounded worry or fear; (3) eagerness.

The second definition states that anxiety is characterized by an exaggerated or unfounded worry or fear. A dental patient's fear is not unfounded, or, indeed exaggerated. We, as dentists, may feel that the fear is unfounded; however, about half the population avoids visiting the dentist due to fear of pain. With the advent of modern dental techniques, this theoretically should not be so. With proper local anesthesia, nitrous oxide/oxygen analgesia and topical anesthesia, why should patients still be frightened? The answer lies partially in the dental profession and partially in the educational background of the individual patient.

In general, human beings do not like to experience pain; in fact, they do not even like to think about pain. They will try to avoid any situation that might prove to be painful. It is difficult to undo prior frightening dental experiences and resultant preconceived notions, but it is vital that we recognize a patient's anxiety and help him deal with it. We must also recognize that differences exist in pain perception. Before describing how to recognize anxiety and the variations in pain perception, it is important to recognize that there is a relation between pain and anxiety which forms a vicious, pain-anxiety cycle. Pain is almost always linked with and potentiated by anxiety. The anxious individual has less tolerance for pain. Pain, in turn, can produce anxiety; anxiety lowers the threshold of pain perception. Questions like, "How long will the pain last?" "Does it mean something serious?" are often thought and even expressed. It is up to the practitioner to try to at least "bend" the pain-anxiety cycle if he cannot break it.

Regular and emergency dental patients undergo varying degrees of physical and psychological stress. The dentist should pay close attention to the verbal and non-verbal signs of fear and anxiety and should regard each individual according to his needs. Some patients need psychological reassurance, others only need to know that enough time is allotted for the local anesthesia to be effective.

If one can accept most complaints as pleas and react accordingly, the dentist will truly feel like the healing practitioner we all should aspire to be.

Several ways to recognize anxiety are:

A. Listen to the vocal tone of the patient as well as to what is said.

B. Observe how the patient positions himself in the chair. Are the eyes shut? Are the fists clenched?

C. Is the person fidgeting? Are the person's eyes moving and looking at all the equipment and instruments?

D. Anxiety is often seen in the questions asked, i.e., "What is this for?"

E. The expression on the patient's face may reveal anxiety.

F. Questions are often used to delay treatment as are frequent drinks of water.

The preceding list is a cursory one, but does illustrate some of the verbal and nonverbal messages conveyed concerning the patient's uneasiness.

Many times the patient's anxiety or uneasiness can be helped by informing the person you are aware of the strain they are undergoing and you are willing to help alleviate the problem.

To project understanding of the patient's problem is at times the best type of psychological support. Other patients may need pretreatment medication for their anxiety such as 2 or 5 mg of Valium taken ½ hour before bedtime and ½ hour before the appointment. Some patients may need nitrous oxide/oxygen analgesia. The point is that the patient should know that there is more than one approach to managing him and his dental problems.

II. Pain Perception

Just as it is important to recognize anxiety in a patient, it is important to understand the variations in pain perception. Since the dawn of civilization pain has been one of humankind's persistent torments. People search for relief by ingesting, injecting or topically applying a variety of medicaments. There is a dual nature to pain perception; first, the physiological and anatomical process by which pain is received and transmitted by neural structures to the central nervous system. The second half is the patient's individual perception of unpleasant experiences. These individual perceptions vary due to personal differences in environment and upbringing, in conjunction with socioeconomic factors and societal conditioning. To understand the personal differences in environment one must realize that no matter how few or how many children exist in a family, the parental influence is different with each child. This difference can depend on family conditions when one child is growing up in contrast to another. There are also differences in the first born, middle and last born children. It is also established that parental relationships vary according to the sex and personality of the individual children. Each has a personal environment in which they grow up. Accordingly, each individual who seeks treatment must be considered a personal and individual human being and treated as such. Unfortunately, this is often not the case. The dentist and other healing practitioners who do not approach people in a supportive manner have helped to establish behavior where people expect to be unhappy and anxious during dental treatment and often "complain" about the most minor procedures.

Some additional factors that have a bearing on a patient's pain reaction threshold are:

A. Emotional Traits

The patient who is emotionally unstable will usually have a low pain threshold. Patients who are greatly concerned or who have problems—not necessarily related to the dental problem—have a low pain threshold.

B. Fatigue

This can be related to the patient who may have been up all night or who had a restless night. At times this can be further complicated by the long waits in the emergency clinic.

C. Age of Patient

Older people tend to tolerate pain better than young people. They achieve a philosophy that unpleasant experiences are a part of life.

D. Sex

There are various theories as to which sex tolerates pain and discomfort better. Some researchers postulate that men seem to tolerate discomfort better as a reflection of man's desire to maintain his feeling of superiority. Most individuals believe pain tolerance relates more to individual differences than sex differences.

E. Fear and Apprehension

The pain threshold is lowered as fear and apprehension rise. People who are apprehensive tend to magnify, within their minds, an "unpleasant" experience. Unpleasantness becomes discomfort, and discomfort becomes pain!

The patient must be listened to, spoken with and given support in order to alleviate apprehension. Procedures should be explained in language that is understandable to the patient and the doctor should avoid being too graphic since the patient can imagine unreal and unwanted experiences. An example of this would be telling a patient, "We are going to take the nerve out of your tooth." The patient can picture a very painful procedure. He visualizes something similar to a live wire being removed, as he knows at times when the dentist is near the "nerve" it can be painful. What must it feel like if the "nerve" is taken out? It is more adequate to state, after appropriate anesthesia, that the area where the nerve is located will be cleaned out. The patient should be reassured that sufficient anesthesia will be given and the proper waiting period observed for the anesthesia to work. In that a local anesthesia is usually given, it should be explained that the patient will feel the pressure of reamers and files because, although the area is "numb," he is not unconscious. At times careful planning can avoid a crisis.

F. Past Experience

Bad past experiences can raise the anxiety and lower the pain threshold; again, with proper preparation and understanding, most people can be helped. The patient must be reassured and motivated.

G. Drugs

Various drugs alter the pain threshold. Narcotics elevate the pain threshold at the central nervous system level. Narcotics can also cause the patient to be calmed or even euphoric; therefore, these agents may alter pain reactions by controlling emotional and psychological factors.

Barbiturates actually lower the pain threshold; however, if the pain perception is controlled, the sedative effect of these drugs may alter the patient's emotional status in such a manner that he can work with his problem better.

Psychosedatives (tranquilizers) actually do not elevate or lower the pain threshold;

however, their ability to relax the patient helps allay the fear and apprehension and therefore can be a valuable adjunct in pain and anxiety control.

III. Patient Stress

From all that has been stated to this point, it is quite obvious that both routine and emergency dental patients, within varying degrees, are undergoing stress, both emotional and physical. Unfortunately, many verbal and nonverbal messages exhibited by dental patients are dismissed or ignored and services are delivered in part to maintain pace with scheduled patients. Emergency patients' pleas may be heeded even less as they may be disrupting the time schedule. The major difference between the stress of routine and emergency patient seems to be the pre- and post-treatment duration of the stress reactions.

Negative emotional states can be considered an indication of stress. A patient displaying fear, anger, depression and, of course, anxiety, can reveal that the patient is undergoing stress.

Often the label "anxiety" is used when the condition is actually fear. A person who is able to receive an injection or have some operative procedure in a moment can exhibit fear; however, if someone fears a contemplated procedure in the distant future this can more appropriately be labeled anxiety.

Other stress indications are changes in motor behavior. Some clues to changes in motor behavior in stress response are: increased muscle tension, disturbances of speech, the facial expressions accompanying speech and how intense the behavior is.

There can also be an alteration in cognitive processes due to stress. Some of the cognitive functions affected can be judgment, memory, problem solving and the normal social interactions that are needed to conduct a therapeutic session. At times stressed patients do not listen well and at times they do not remember instructions.

There are physiologic indications of stress. Some of the better known autonomic changes accompanying stress responses are: increased heart rate, increased respiration and sweat gland activity.

Epinephrine from the adrenal medulla produces some of the aforementioned changes as well as other actions in the gastrointestinal tract and brain. The adrenal cortex can be stimulated by stress of physical or mental origins. This produces corticosteroids which can have effects on the physiology and psychology of the patient. Physical pain, tissue damage and use of local anesthetic drugs are capable of causing the release of increased quantities of free corticosteroids from the adrenal cortex. At times, when a patient is awaiting dental local anesthesia, an elevation in the level of corticosteroids may result. It is therefore difficult to judge whether a physiologic stress reaction was induced by the anesthetic or by psychologically anticipating the injection.

The extent of this psychological reaction is dependent upon the level of anxiety or fear the patient has in conjunction with the methods of management that he is receiving from the dentist. Emergency patients would seem to need more support in order to alleviate the stress they are under due to some problems. There are indications that there is greater incidence of syncope in emergency patients than in nonemergency patients.

IV. Categories of Dental Patients

It seems necessary to form a separate classification in order to understand emergency patients. Although it is unwise to place human beings in "pigeon holes," it can be helpful when treating an emergency patient to understand some of the psychodynamics. The categories, which are extremely broad (and certainly can be further subdivided), are:

A. Emergency Person with a Dental Problem

1. Hostile
2. Cooperative

B. Dental Patient with a Dental Problem

1. Cooperative
2. Hostile
3. Irregular

The categories have been so delineated as to differentiate people who function on an emergency level only (emergency person with a dental problem) and those patients who receive dental care but now have a special problem.

A. Emergency Person with a Dental Problem

1. Hostile. The emergency person with a dental problem will no more go for prophylactic routine dental visits than he would go to an orthopedist to check his bone structure. The pain extraction cycle has not been broken. They can be extremely anxious and hostile. A subcategory of this class behaves this way due to fear and ignorance of dental procedures. There can be a gross injection phobia and fear of any doctor. There can be a total lack of dental hygiene and motivation for care due to many other factors. At times they will not accept responsibility for their problems—the dentist is a person they must see "who will hurt" them while they are "already hurting." They are "professional clinic patients" who accept waiting and shifting to different departments; however, in the course of the "accepted" waiting, the overt anxiety grows as does the often overt hostility. These individuals are extremely difficult to motivate for regular or irregular care. However, if an interest is shown in them and their anxious questions are answered, some can be motivated to improve their dental outlook and possibly receive more than the automatic extraction.

2. Cooperative. Many of the educational factors of this individual are the same as for the hostile emergency person. They lack the same dental education and/or motivation. A basic difference is that they accept their plight as a part of "normal life" and are cooperative when receiving treatment. They are easier to motivate for limited care, but often do not have the desire or finances to continue with their care. Obviously, they too are "professional clinic patients" and totally accept the waiting, etc. The basic difference between them and their hostile counterpart is that they recognize their responsibility for their pain even if it is due to neglect and do not view the dentist as a person who is part of the cause of their discomfort. Even though they usually do not see a dentist except when in pain, they will occasionally report to a dentist for extraction when they are in severe pain because a tooth "broke" or has become loose. The fear is not as great as it is in the emergency patient who is hostile and they will avoid getting a toothache when they have received a warning. They fear dental procedures, but to a small extent fear the sequela of total neglect also.

If a supportive approach is used and a realistic treatment proposed (that is, a treatment plan within the emotional, financial and psychological reach of the patient), this unfortunate individual will accept at least some preventative and restorative procedures.

B. Dental Patient with a Dental Problem

1. Cooperative. This type of patient is by far the most cooperative and simplest to manage. They receive regular care but something has gone "wrong." Depending on past dental experience and their relationship with the treating dentist, they make it all "easy." Fortunately for all practicing dentists, the greater percentage of routine patients is this type of individual. This does not mean that they should be taken for granted; in fact, they should receive support and interest in order to help them continue as they are.

2. Hostile. Some dental patients with a dental problem can be the most hostile of all. The hostility can be manifested in a covert manner. Subtle barbs and messages are relayed. Basically, there are several items that are upsetting them. Something that they paid for has gone wrong, the discomfort they are having is the dentist's fault and they are spending time taking care of the problem. In order to treat this type of individual, it is necessary not to be on the defensive. Limits must be set. All procedures must be clearly defined so as to avoid ambiguity. It is not unusual for them to state, "Oh, another x-ray" or "more red tape," etc. The practitioner must be assertive and positive without being aggressive or defensive. Often the doctor's professional judgment is questioned concerning a restoration that broke or tooth structure that broke out with the restoration. While it may be difficult, the problem should be explained; appear sure of yourself and don't be intimidated, and these patients, too, will be treatable.

3. Irregular Care. This category of patient, which is quite large, does not have regular maintenance visits. They will have restorative work done when an emergency arises in addition to nonregular care which may transpire every two or three years.

This patient usually doesn't exhibit fear or apprehension but does not place a great value on oral health. The administering of treatment is usually easy but they are hard to motivate for full care. The loss of a tooth here or there is not that important to them. If they are approached with a practical treatment plan that they can afford, they will go through episodes of regular care. They recognize their personal responsibility for the emergency; therefore, they cooperate while being treated.

Drugs Most Often Used in Dentistry and Common Drug Interactions

LEVENTE Z. BODAK-GYOVAI

Analgesics

Non-Narcotic Analgesics (use p.r.n., q.i.d.)
Tylenol (acetaminophen) 325 mg tab.
Aspirin (acetylsalicylic acid) 325 mg tab.
Ponstel Kapseals (mefenamic acid) 500 mg initial, 250 mg.
Synalgos (phenacetin, aspirin, promethazine, caffeine) caps.
Empirin Compound (aspirin, phenacetin, caffeine).
Fiorinal (butalbital, caffeine, aspirin, phenacetin) caps., tab.
Darvon Compound (phenacetin, propoxyphene, aspirin, caffeine) pulvules.
Darvacet-N 100 (propoxyphene, acetaminophen) tab.
Darvon-N with ASA (propoxyphene, aspirin) tab.
Norgesic (orphenadrine, aspirin, phenacetin, caffeine) tab.
Norgesic Forte is twice the strength of Norgesic.

Strong Narcotic Analgesics (use p.r.n., t.i.d. or q.i.d.)
Empirin with codeine (No. 1 = 7.5 mg codeine, No. 2 = 15 mg codeine, No. 3 = 30 mg codeine, No. 4 = 60 mg codeine; aspirin) tab.

Fiorinal with codeine (No. 1 = 7.5 mg codeine, No. 2 = 15 mg codeine, No. 3 = 30 mg codeine; butalbital, caffeine, aspirin, phenacetin).

Phenaphen with codeine (No. 2 = 15 mg codeine, No. 3 = 30 mg codeine, No. 4 = 60 mg; acetaminophen) caps.

Tylenol with codeine (No. 1 = 7.5 mg codeine, No. 2 = 15 mg codeine, No. 3 = 30 mg codeine, No. 4 = 60 codeine; acetaminophen) tab.

Dilaudid (dihydromorphinone or hydromorphone) 1, 2, 3 or 4 mg tab.
Percodan (oxycodone 4.9 mg, aspirin, caffeine, phenacetin) tab.
Percodan-Demi (oxycodone 2.45 mg, aspirin, caffeine, phenacetin) tab.
Demerol (meperidine) 50, 100 mg tab. and 2 ml cartridges (50 mg per 1 ml) IM.
Pantopon (alkaloids of opium) adult dose 20 mg per 1 ml amp. IM, SC.
Nisentil (alphaprodine) 40 mg per 1 ml amp. IM.
Demerol 2 ml cartridges (50 mg per 1 ml) IM.

Narcotic Antagonist
Narcan (naloxone) dose: 0.4 mg per 1 ml IV, IM, SC.

Sedative-Hypnotic Analgesics

Non-Barbiturates
Phenergan (promethazine) 12.5, 25 mg tab. and 25 mg per 1 ml amp. IM.
Atarax (hydroxyzine) 10, 25, 50, 100 mg tab.
Vistaril (hydroxyzine) 25, 50, 100 mg caps.

Barbiturates
Amytal (amobarbital) 15, 30, 50 mg tab. and 65 mg per amp. IV, IM.
Luminal (phenobarbital) 16, 32 mg tab.
Nembutal (pentobarbital) 30, 50, 100 mg caps.

Seconal (secobarbital) 30, 50, 100 mg pulvules.

Sedative-Analgesic Combination
Mepergan (50 mg Demerol, 12.5 mg Phenergan) caps.
Mepergan Fortis (50 mg Demerol, 25 mg Phenergan) caps.

Antianxiety Agents
Librium (chlordiazepoxide) 5, 10, 25 mg. caps.
Libritabs (chlordiazepoxide) 5, 10, 25 mg, tab.
Valium (diazepam) 2, 5, 10 mg, tab.
Vistaril (hydroxyzine) 25, 50, 100 mg, caps.

Tricyclic Antidepressants
Tofranil (imipramine) 10, 25, 50 mg tab. 75, 100, 125, 150 mg caps.
Sinequan (doxepin) 10, 25, 50, 75, 100, 150 mg caps.
Elavil (amitriptyline) 10, 25, 75, 100, 150 mg tab.

Antibiotics

Penicillin
Penicillin G 125, 250 mg tab.
Wycillin IM. Procaine.
Bicillin L-A IM. Benzathine.
Amcill (ampicillin) 250, 500 mg caps, chewable, 125, 250 mg susp.
Pen-Vee-K (phenoxymethyl penicillin) 125, 250, 500 mg tab.
Penicillin V 250, 500 mg tabs. 125, 250 mg susp.
V-Cillin-K 125, 250, 500 mg tabs.
Tegopen (cloxacillin) 250, 500 mg caps.
Ampicillin 250, 500 mg caps., 125, 250 mg susp.
Amoxicillin (Polymox, Amoxil, Larotid) 250, 500 mg caps., 125, 250 mg susp.
Polycillin (ampicillin) 250, 500 mg caps., 125 mg tab., chewable 125, 250, 500 mg susp.
Principen (ampicillin) 250, 500 mg caps., 125, 250 mg susp.

Erythromycin
Erythromycin stearate 250, 500 mg tab.
E-Mycin 250 mg tab.
Erythromycin 250 mg enteric coated tab.
E.E.S. 200 mg chewable., 200, 400 mg tab. (erythrocin ethyl succinate)
Ilosone (erythromycin estolate) 125, 250 mg caps, 125, 250 mg tab. chewable 125, 250 mg susp.

Tetracycline
Achromycin (tetracycline) 100, 250, 500 mg caps.
Cyclopar (tetracycline) 250, 500 mg caps.
Sumycin (tetracycline) 250, 500 mg caps.
Aureomycin (chlortetracycline) 250 mg caps.
Terramycin (oxytetracycline) 125, 250 mg caps.
Minocin (minocycline) 50, 100 mg caps.
Vibramycin (doxycycline) 50, 100 mg caps.

Tetracyclines in Combination with Antifungal Drug
Achrostatin-V (tetracycline, nystatin) caps.
Terrastatin (oxytetracycline, nystatin) caps.
Mysteclin-F (tetracycline, amphotericin B) caps.

Other
Keflex (cephalexin) 250, 500 mg pulvules, caps.
Cleocin (clindamycin) 75, 150 mg caps.
Lincocin (lincomycin) 500 mg caps.
Velosef (cephrodine) 250, 500 mg caps., 125, 250 mg susp.

Antifungal Agents
Mycostatin (nystatin) ointment, vaginal tab., oral susp., oral tab.
Fungizone (amphotericin B) ointment.
Griseofulvin Microsize 125, 250, 500 mg tab.

Local Anesthetics with or without Vasoconstrictor for Infiltration and Block
AMIDES:
Xylocaine (lidocaine).
Carbocaine (mepivacaine).
Citanest (prilocaine).
Marcaine (bupivacaine).

ESTERS:
Monocaine (butethamine).
Primacaine (metabutoxycaine).
Cyclaine (hexylcaine).
Metycaine (piperocaine).
Unacaine (metabutethamine).
Ravocaine (propoxycaine).

For Surface Anesthesia
AMIDES:
Nupercaine (dibucaine).
Xylocaine (lidocaine).

ESTERS:
Benzocaine (ethyl aminobenzoate).
Butyn (butacaine).
Pontocaine (tetracaine).

OTHER:
Benadryl (diphenhydramine).
Dyclone (dyclonine).

General Analgesics—Anesthetics

Inhalation
Nitrous oxide.
Fluothane (halothane).
Vinethene (vinyl ether).

IV
Pentothal (thiopental).
Brevital (methohexital).

Anticholinergic
Atropine 0.4 mg tab.

Antiemetic
Tigan (trimethobenzamide) 100, 250 mg caps, 100 mg pediatric, 200 mg suppository
Compazine (prochlorperazine) 5, 10 mg tab.
Phenergan (promethazine) 25, 50 mg per 1 ml amp. IM, IV.

Corticosteroids for Topical Use
Orabase HCA (hydrocortisone) paste.
Kenalog in Orabase (triamcinolone) emolient.

Vasoconstrictors
Epinephrine (adrenalin).
Levophed (levarterenol).
Neo-Synephrine (phenylephrine).
Note: food interferes with the absorption of per os medications, primarily antibiotics, therefore, the drug should be administered one hour before or two hours after meals.

Table 1
Table of Drug Interactions

Drug Given by Dentist	Drug Taken by Patient	Possible Drug Interaction
Acetaminophen	Anticoagulants	Increased anticoagulant effect
	Antihypertensives	Increased antihypertensive effect, CNS depression
	Phenobarbital	Methemoglobinemia
Acetylsalicylic acid	Alcohol	Gastric purpura
	Anticoagulants	Increased anticoagulant effect
	Barbiturates	Decreased acetylsalicylic acid effect
	Codeine	Increased analgesic effect
	Diphenylhydantoin	Increased effect of diphenylhydantoin
	Furosemide	Toxic effect of acetylsalicylic acid
	Imipramin	Can be lethal
	Indomethacin	Decreased anti-inflammatory effect of indomethacin, aggravate peptic ulcer
	Oral antidiabetics	Increased hypoglycemic effect
	Penicillin	Increased penicillin effect
	Phenobarbital	Decreased analgesic effect of acetylsalicylic acid
	Phenothiazines	Increased CNS depression
	Phenylbutazone	Decreased anti-inflammatory effect of phenylbutazone
	Propoxyphene	Increased analgesia
Alphaprodine	Alcohol	Increased CNS depression
	Analgesics	Increased analgesia
	Anesthetics	Increased CNS depression
	Anticholinergics	Increased anticholinergic effect, aggravate glaucoma
	Barbiturates	Increased CNS depression
	Chlorpromazine	Increased CNS depression
	MAO inhibitors	Paresthesia, hypotension
	Penicillin	Increased penicillin effect
	Phenobarbital	Decreased analgesic effect

Table 1— *Continued*

Drug Given by Dentist	Drug Taken by Patient	Possible Drug Interaction
	Phenothiazines	Increased CNS depressions
	Sulfonamides	Increased sulfonamide effect
Amitriptyline	Alcohol	Increased CNS depression
	Antidepressants	Mutual potentiation effect
	Chlordiazepoxide	Increased CNS depression
	Methyldopa	Hypertension, tachycardia
	MAO inhibitors	Seizures, can be lethal
	Reserpine	Hypertension
Amobarbital (see Barbiturates)		
Amphotericin B	Cardiac glycosides	Digitalis toxicity due to hypokalemia caused by amphotericin B
	Muscle relaxants	Toxic effect of muscle relaxants due to hypokalemia caused by amphotericin B
Ampicillin (see Penicillin)		
Atropine	Acetylcholine	Decreased effect of acetylcholine
	Chlorpromazine	Increased atropine effect
	Isoniazid	Increased atropine effect, aggravate glaucoma
	MAO inhibitors	Increased atropine effect
	Meperidine	Mutually increased effects
	Phenothiazines	Mutually increased effects, aggravate glaucoma
	Reserpine	Mutually decreased effects
	Tricyclic antidepressants	Increased atropine effect
Barbiturates	Acidifying beverages	Increased barbiturate effect
	Alcohol	Increased CNS depression
	Alkalinizing substances	Decreased barbiturate effect
	Aminopyrine	Mutually decreased effect
	Analgesics	Decreased effect of mild analgesics, increased CNS depression of narcotic analgesics
	Anesthetics	Increased CNS depression
	Anticonvulsants	Decreased anticonvulsant effect
	Antidepressants	Mutually increased effect
	Antihistamines	Early increased CNS depression, late mutual inhibition
	Anti-inflammatory agents	Decreased anti-inflammatory effect
	Ascorbic acid	Increased barbiturate effect
	Chlordiazepoxide	Increased CNS depression
	Chlorpromazine	Increased sedative effect
	CNS depressants (alcohol, barbiturates, narcotics, phenothiazines, etc.)	Increased CNS depression, can be fatal
	Corticosteroids	Decreased steroid effect
	Diazepam	Increased CNS depression
	Diphenhydramine	Mutual inhibition
	Diphenylhydantoin	Decreased anticonvulsant effect
	Hydroxyzine	Increased barbiturate effect
	MAO inhibitors	Increased barbiturate effect
	Meprobamate	Increased CNS depression
	Minor tranquilizers	Increased CNS depression

Table 1— *Continued*

Drug Given by Dentist	Drug Taken by Patient	Possible Drug Interaction
	Oral anticoagulants	Decreased anticoagulant effect, increased barbiturate effect
	Oral antidiabetics	Mutually increased effects
	Oral contraceptives	Decreased contraceptive effect
	Phenacetin	Decreased phenacetin effect
	Phenothiazines	Increased CNS depression
	Phenylbutazone	Decreased phenylbutazone effect
	Reserpine	Hypotension, bradycardia
	Sodium bicarbonate	Decreased barbiturate effect
	Salicylates	Decreased salicylate effect
	Sulfonamides	Decreased sulfonamide effect
	Thiazide diuretics	Orthostatic hypotension
	Thyroid preparations	Decreased barbiturate effect
Bupivacaine (see Local Anesthestics)		
Butacaine (see Local Anesthetics)		
Butalbital (see Barbiturates)		
Butethamine (see Local Anesthetics)		
Cephalexin	Penicillins	Increased antibacterial effect, cross-resistance, cross-sensitivity
Chlordiazepoxide	Alcohol	Increased CNS depression
	Anticoagulants	Decreased anticoagulant effect
	Barbiturates	Increased CNS depression
	CNS depressants	Mutually increased effects
	Codeine	Coma
	Diazepam	Urinary incontinence
	MAO inhibitors	Increased chlordiazepoxide effects
	Narcotics	Hypotension
	Phenothiazines	Increased CNS depression
	Tricyclic antidepressants	Mutually increased effects
Chlortetracycline (see Tetracyclines)		
Clindamycin	Opiates, atropine	Aggravate colitis
	Neuromuscular blocking agents	Increased effect of neuromuscular agents
Cloxacillin (see Penicillins)		
Caffeine	Anticoagulants	Decreased anticoagulant effect
	Sympathomimetics	Increased CNS stimulation
	Xanthines	Increased CNS stimulation
Corticosteroids	Anticholinergics	Aggravate glaucoma
	Anticonvulsants	Decreased steroid effect
	Antidiabetics	Decreased antidiabetic effect
	Antihistamines	Decreased steroid effect
	Barbiturates	Decreased steroid effect, increased sedative effect
	Digitalis	Hypokalemia, digitalis toxicity

Table 1— *Continued*

Drug Given by Dentist	Drug Taken by Patient	Possible Drug Interaction
	Diphenhydramine	Decreased steroid effect
	Diphenylhydantoin	Decreased steroid effect
	Diuretics	Hypokalemia
	General anesthetics	Profound hypotension
	Meperidine	Aggravate glaucoma
	Oral anticoagulants	Decreased anticoagulant effect
	Phenylbutazone	Decreased steroid effect
	Propranolol	Decreased steroid effect
	Salicylates	Increased anti-inflammatory effect
	Sympathomimetics	Aggravate glaucoma
	Tricyclic antidepressants	Aggravate glaucoma
Diazepam	Alcohol	Hypotension, increased CNS depression
	Anticonvulsants	Decreased anticonvulsant effect
	Antihypertensives	Increased antihypertensive effect
	Barbiturates	Increased CNS depression
	Caffeine	Decreased diazepam effect
	CNS depressants	Increased CNS depression
	MAO inhibitors	Increased diazepam effect
	Tricyclic antidepressants	Increased diazepam effect
Dibucaine (see Local Anesthetics)		
Dihydromorphinone (hydromorphone)		
Diphenhydramine	Alcohol	Increased CNS depression
	Anticoagulants	Decreased anticoagulant effect
	Atropine	Increased atropine effects
	Barbiturates	Mutually decreased effects
	CNS depressants	Increased CNS depression
	Corticosteroids	Decreased steroid effects
	Diphenylhydantoin	Mutually decreased effects
	Epinephrine	Increased epinephrine effects
	MAO inhibitors	Increased diphenhydramine effects
	Norepinephrine	Increased norepinephrine effect
	Phenylbutazone	Mutually decreased effect
Dyclonine		
Epinephrine	Alcohol	Decreased epinephrine effect
	Alpha adrenergic blockers	Hypotension (epinephrine reversal)
	Antidiabetics	Decreased antidiabetic effect
	Antihistamines	Increased epinephrine effect
	Chlorpromazine	Hypotension (epinephrine reversal)
	Digitalis glycosides	Cardiac arrhythmias
	Ephedrine	Increased epinephrine effects
	General anesthetics	Cardiac arrhythmias
	Isoproterenol	Cardiac arrhythmias
	MAO inhibitors	Hypertension
	Mephentermine	Hypertension
	Miotics	Glaucoma
	Nitrates and nitrites	Hypotension
	Phenothiazines	Hypotension
	Phenylephrine	Hypertension
	Sympathomimetics	Hypertension, can be lethal

Table 1— *Continued*

Drug Given by Dentist	Drug Taken by Patient	Possible Drug Interaction
	Thyroid preparations (hormones)	Coronary insufficiency
	Tricyclic antidepressants	Increased epinephrine effects

Note: Epinephrine is contraindicated in hyperthyroid patients, in cardiac patients (doses over 0.2 mg) and in those who are on guanethidine or reserpine-like adrenergic blockers.

Drug Given by Dentist	Drug Taken by Patient	Possible Drug Interaction
Erythromycin	Acidifying beverages	Decreased erythromycin effect
	Lincomycin	Mutually antagonistic effects
	Penicillins	Decreased erythromycin effect
Ethyl aminobenzoate (see Local Anesthetics)		
Halothane	Epinephrine	Tachycardia, fibrillation, cardiac stand-still
	Mephentermine	Cardiac arrhythmias
	Nitrous oxide	Hypotension, bradycardia
	Nordefrin	Cardiac arrhythmias
	Norepinephrine	Tachycardia, fibrillation, cardiac stand-still
Hexylcaine (see Local Anesthetics)		
Hydrocortisone (see Corticosteroids)		
Hydroxyzine	Alcohol	Increased CNS depression
	Barbiturates	Increased CNS depression
	CNS depressants	Increased CNS depression
	Heparin	Decreased anticoagulant effect
	Oral anticoagulants	Increased anticoagulant effect
Levarterenol	Alcohol	Decreased levarterenol effect
	Amphetamines	Increased levarterenol effect
	Antihistamines	Increased levarterenol effect
	General anesthetics	Tachycardia, fibrillation, can be lethal
	MAO inhibitors	Hypertension, tachycardia, coma (hypertensive crisis)
	Methyldopa	Hypertension
	Nitrous oxide	Hypertension
	Reserpine	Aggravate bronchial asthma
	Thyroid preparations	Coronary insufficiency
	Tricyclic antidepressants	Increased levarterenol effect
Lidocaine (see Local Anesthetics)		
Lincomycin	Antidiarrheals	Decreased lincomycin effect
	Erythromycin	Mutually decreased effects
Local anesthetics	Cardiovascular depressants	Increased cardiovascular depression
	CNS depressants	Increased CNS depression
	Procainamide	CNS stimulation, restlessness, hallucinations
	Sulfonamides	Decreased sulfonamide effect

Table 1—_Continued_

Drug Given by Dentist	Drug Taken by Patient	Possible Drug Interaction
Meperidine	Amphetamine	Increased meperidine effect
	Atropine	Aggravate glaucoma
	Corticosteroids	Aggravate glaucoma
	General anesthetics	Hypotension
	MAO inhibitors	Increased CNS depression (hypertension, convulsions, coma, death)
	Nitrates, nitrites	Hypotension
	Oral contraceptives	Increased meperidine effect
	Phenobarbital	Early increased, late decreased meperidine effect
	Phenothiazines	Increased CNS depression, can be lethal
	Tricyclic antidepressants	Aggravate glaucoma, increased respiratory depression
Mefenamic acid		
Mepivacaine (see Local Anesthetics)		
Metabutethamine (see Local Anesthetics)		
Metabutoxycaine (see Local Anesthetics)		
Methohexital (see Barbiturates)		
Naloxone	Narcotics	Reversed narcotic effect
Nitrous oxide	Halothane	Hypotension, bradycardia
	Norepinephrine	Hypertension
Nystatin		
Opium	Alcohol	Increased CNS depression
	Analeptics	Convulsions
	CNS depressants	Increased CNS depression, coma, death
	Diuretics	Orthostatic hypotension
	MAO inhibitors	Increased narcotic analgesic effect
	Oral anticoagulants	Increased anticoagulant effect
	Pentazocine	Decreased narcotic analgesic effect
	Phenothiazines	Increased phenothiazine effect
	Propranolol	Increased morphine effect
	Tricyclic antidepressants	Increased CNS depression
Orphenadrine	Aminopyrine	Decreased aminopyrine effect
	Chlorpromazine	Hypoglycemia, coma
	Hexobarbital	Decreased hexobarbital effect
	Phenylbutazone	Decreased phenylbutazone effect
Oxycodone (see Opium)		
Oxytetracycline (see Tetracycline)		
Penicillins	Acetylsalicylic acid	Increased penicillin effect
	Acidifying beverages	Decreased penicillin effect
	Alkalinizing substances	Decreased penicillin effect

Table 1— *Continued*

Drug Given by Dentist	Drug Taken by Patient	Possible Drug Interaction
	Analgesics	Increased penicillin effect
	Antacids	Decreased penicillin effect
	Anticoagulants	Increased anticoagulant effect (except heparin)
	Blue cheese	Decreased penicillin effect
	Cephalosporins	Cross-resistance, increased antibacterial effect, cross-sensitivity
	Chloramphenicol	Decreased penicillin effect
	Erythromycin	Decreased penicillin effect, except *Staphylococcus aureus*
	Heparin	Decreased anticoagulant effect
	Sulfonamides	Decreased penicillin effect
	Tetracyclines	Decreased penicillin effect
Pentobarbital (see Barbiturates)		
Phenacetin	Phenobarbital	Decreased phenacetin effect
Phenobarbital (see Barbiturates)		
Phenothiazines	Acetylsalicylic acid	Increased CNS depression
	Alcohol	Increased CNS depression
	Analgesics	Increased CNS depression
	Anesthetics	Increased CNS depression
	Anticoagulants	Decreased anticoagulant effect
	Anticonvulsants	Decreased anticonvulsant effect
	Antihistamines	Increased CNS depression
	Antihypertensives	Increased antihypertensive effect
	Barbiturates	Increased sedative effect
	Chlordiazepoxide	Increased CNS depression
	CNS depressants	Increased CNS depression
	Diazepam	Increased CNS depression
	MAO inhibitors	Mutually increased effects
	Minor tranquilizers	Increased CNS depression
	Oral antidiabetics	Increased antidiabetic effect
	Oral contraceptives	Increased phenothiazine effect
	Reserpine	Increased CNS depression
	Sulfonamides	Increased sulfonamide effect
	Thiazide diuretics	Hypotension
	Tricyclic antidepressants	Increased CNS depression

Note: Epinephrine with phenothiazines may result in epinephrine reversal.

Phenylephrine	Epinephrine	Cardiac arrhythmias, acute hypertensive crisis
	Halothane	Cardiac arrhythmias
	MAO inhibitors	Acute hypertensive crisis
Piperocaine (see Local Anesthetics)		
Prilocaine (see Local Anesthetics)		
Promethazine (see Phenothiazines)		

Table 1— *Continued*

Drug Given by Dentist	Drug Taken by Patient	Possible Drug Interaction
Propoxyphene	Acetylsalicylic acid	Increased analgesia
	Alcohol	Increased CNS depression
	Analeptics (amphetamine, caffeine)	Fatal convulsions
	Orphenadrine	Tremor, anxiety, confusion
Secobarbital (see Barbiturates)		
Tetracaine (see Local Anesthetics)		
Tetracycline	Acidifying beverages	Increased tetracycline effect
	Aminopyrine	Increased aminopyrine effect
	Alcohol	Increased tetracycline effect
	Alkalinizing beverages	Decreased tetracycline effect
	Antacids	Decreased tetracycline effect
	Anticoagulants	Increased anticoagulant effect
	Barbiturates	Increased barbiturate effect
	Calcium	Decreased tetracycline effect
	Iron	Decreased tetracycline effect
	Penicillins	Decreased penicillin effect
Thiopental (see Barbiturates)		
Triamcinolone (see Corticosteroids)		
Trimethobenzamide	CNS depressants	Convulsions, coma

appendix
3

Viewing Radiographs Correctly

ROBERT BEIDEMAN

Interpreting radiographs accurately involves coordination of knowledge and experience skills in order to synthesize a diagnosis.

The viewer's first responsibility is to determine the acceptability of the radiographs from a technical aspect. If the films do not cover the areas in question without distortion from such factors as excessive elongation, foreshortening, cone cutting or film bending, they should not be used. Insisting that radiographs be technically acceptable is a prerequisite to accurate interpretation.

It is important to establish a systematic approach when examining radiographs. No single method or system is better than another as long as all information on the radiographs is considered. Large areas of disease attract eye attention and may cause the viewer to overlook other, more subtle, pathologic changes. Systematic viewing will eliminate this problem. It is suggested that when viewing dental radiographs each tooth surface, the peridontium and the bony architecture be examined separately.

In general, radiographs should be viewed with subdued background light. A viewbox with even light distribution over the opaque surface and preferably a rheostat to vary the light intensity is important. Holding x-rays up to a ceiling light or outside light through a window does not give even light intensity because the eye is distracted by surrounding extraneous objects. A viewbox focuses attention on the radiographs in question. The radiographs should be mounted to further exclude background light and relieve eye fatigue. A variable intensity light source within the viewbox can often accentuate subtle density changes otherwise not discernible. A very high intensity light source, such as a bare light bulb, is often useful to view an area on a radiograph when the film is too dark. Overly dark radiographs have much information on them and require only a light source strong enough to visualize them clearly. Overly light radiographs do not contain much information and cannot be "doctored up" to bring out concealed information. A magnifying glass should always be near at hand. Magnification has been proven to enhance small detail changes. Magnification also focuses direct attention of the eyes on very specific areas within a radiograph. All too frequently, the viewer's eye takes in a periapical film in its entirety when many specific areas within the film should be viewed.

This leads to the final point in proper viewing of radiographs. The film should be viewed from near and far. The adage of not seeing the forest for the trees and the trees for the forest is true. Viewing a full-mouth series of radiographs from two or three feet away will point out general areas of radiopacity and radiolucency within the bony architecture and should lead the viewer's eye into a systematic approach of close-up examination of the "trees within the forest."

Following these basic principles when

181

viewing radiographs should lead to a more accurate assessment of the information contained on the film. Correlation of this information with patient history, clinical examination and laboratory studies will aid the clinician in establishing a final diagnosis based on the maximum use of the information available.

References

Ackerman, L.V., Rosai, J. *Surgical Pathology*, Ed. 5. C.V. Mosby Co., St. Louis, 1974.

Alfano, M.C., DeFaola, D.P. Symposium on nutrition. *Dent. Clin. North Am.,* 20(3):461–472, 549–633, 1976.

Anderson, W.A., Scotti, T.M. *Synopsis of Pathology*, Ed. 8. C.V. Mosby Co., St. Louis, 1972.

Ballinger, W., Rutherford, R., Zuidema, G. *The Management of Trauma*. W.B. Saunders Co., Philadelphia, 1973.

Beeson, P.B., McDermott, W. *Cecil-Loeb Textbook of Medicine*, Ed. 14. W.B. Saunders Co., Philadelphia, 1975.

Bennett, C.R. *Monhein's Local Anesthesia and Pain Control in Dental Practice*. C.V. Mosby Co., St. Louis, 1974.

Bennett, C.R. *General Anesthesia in Dental Practice*. C.V. Mosby Co., St. Louis, 1974.

Bennett, C.R. *Conscious Sedation in Dental Practice*. C.V. Mosby Co., St. Louis, 1974.

Bental, E., Pillar, T. Symptoms and diseases accompanying arteriosclerotic cerebrovascular events. *Geriatrics*, 27:142–146, 1972.

Berlove, I.J. *Dental-Medical Emergencies and Complications*, Ed. 2. Year Book Medical Publishers, Chicago, 1959.

Best, C., Taylor, N. *The Physiological Basis of Medical Practice*. Williams & Wilkins, Baltimore, 1966.

Bordley, J., Harvey, M. *Differential Diagnosis*. W.B. Saunders Co., Philadelphia, 1972.

Bottomley, W.K. The importance of a detailed drug history for the dentist. *U.S. Nav. Med.*, 62:18, 1973.

Boyd, W. *An Introduction to the Study of Disease*, Ed. 6. Lea and Febiger, Philadelphia, 1974.

Braverman, I.M. *Skin Signs of Systemic Disease*. W.B. Saunders Co., Philadelphia, 1970.

Brook, R.H. A study of the methodologic problem associated with assessment of quality of care. Thesis. The Johns Hopkins University, School of Hygiene and Public Health, Baltimore, 1972.

Burch, C.E. Arterial hypertension and the dental patient. *J. Am. Dent. Assoc.*, 73:102, 1966.

Burch, G.E. *A Primer of Cardiology*, Ed. 4. Lea and Febiger, Philadelphia, 1973.

Burket, L.W. *Oral Medicine: Diagnosis and Treatment*, Ed. 6. J.B. Lippincott Co., Philadelphia, 1971.

Burnside, J.W. *Adam's Physical Diagnosis, An Introduction to Clinical Medicine*, Ed. 15. Williams & Wilkins, Baltimore, 1974.

Cecil, R.L., Loeb, R.F. *Textbook of Medicine*, Ed. 8. W.B. Saunders Co., Philadelphia, 1951.

Chamberlin, F.C. Management of medical-dental problems in patients with cardiovascular diseases. *Mod. Concepts Cardiovasc. Dis.*, 30:697, 1961.

Chatton, M.J., Krupp, M.A. *Current Diagnosis and Treatment*. Lange Medical Publications, Los Altos, Calif., 1972.

Christakis, G. *Nutritional Assessment in Health Programs*. American Public Health Association, Washington, D.C., 1973.

De Nicola, P., Morsiani, M., Zavagli, G. *Nail Disease in International Medicine*. Charles C Thomas, Publishers, Springfield, Ill., 1974.

Dunn, M.J., Booth, D.F. *Dental Auxiliary*. Williams & Wilkins, Baltimore, 1975.

Durham, R.H. *Encyclopedia of Medical Symptoms*. Harper and Row, New York, 1960.

Dworitin, S.F. Psychodynamics of dental emergencies. *Dent. Clin. North Am.*, 17(3):403–416, 1973.

Eastman, R.D. *Biochemical Values in Clinical Medicine*, Ed. 5. Williams & Wilkins, Baltimore, 1975.

Fairbairn, J.F., Juergens, J.L., Spittell, J.A. *Allen, Barker, Aines' Peripheral Vascular Diseases*, Ed. 4. W.B. Saunders Co., Philadelphia, 1972.

Fraizer, C.A. *Dentistry and the Allergic Patient*. Charles C Thomas, Publishers, Springfield, Ill., 1973.

Freedman, G.L., Hooley, J.R. Medical contraindications to the extraction of teeth. *Dent. Clin. North Am.*, 13:939, 1969.

Freis, E.D. The treatment of hypertension. *Am. J. Med.*, 52:664, 1972.

Fröhlich, E.D., Tarazi, R.C., Dustan, H.P. Re-examination of the hemodynamics of hypertension. *Am. J. Med. Sci.*, 257:9–23, 1969.

Gardner, A.F. *Differential Oral Diagnosis in Systemic Disease.* John Wright and Sons, Bristol, England, 1970.

Garg, S. *Laboratory Tests in Common Use*, Ed. 5. Springer Publishing Co., New York, 1971.

Gefter, W.I., Pator, B.H., Myerson, R.M. *Synopsis of Cardiology.* C.V. Mosby Co., St. Louis, 1965.

Glass, R.T., Abla, M., Wheathy, J. Teaching self-examination of the head and neck—another aspect of preventive dentistry. *J. Am. Dent. Assoc.*, 90:1265, 1975.

Goodhart, R.A., Snils, M.E. *Modern Nutrition in Health and Disease*, Ed. 5. Lea and Febiger, Philadelphia, 1973.

Gorlin, R.J., Goldman, M.M. *Thoma's Oral Pathology*, Ed. 6. C.V. Mosby Co., St. Louis, 1970.

Graban, J.C., Kaufman, S., Uthman, A.A., Scott, S.J. A public education program in self-examination for orofacial cancer. *J. Am. Dent. Assoc.*, 96:480, 1978.

Gross, M. Diurnal blood pressure variations in cerebrovascular disease. *Ann. Intern. Med.*, 72:823, 1970.

Halsted, J.A. *The Laboratory in Clinical Medicine.* W.B. Saunders Co., Philadelphia, 1976.

Hamilton, M., Pickering, G.W., Roberts, J.A.F., Sowry, G.S.C. The aetiology of essential hypertension: The arterial pressure in general population. *Clin. Sci.*, 13:11, 1954a.

Hamilton, M., Pickering, G.W., Roberts, J.A.F., Sowry, G.S.C. The aetiology of essential hypertension: Scores for arterial blood pressure adjusted for differences in age and sex. *Clin. Sci.*, 13:87, 1954b.

Harvey, J., Ross, O. *Principles and Practice of Internal Medicine.* Appleton-Century-Crofts, New York, 1972.

Hickler, R.B., Vandam, L.D. Hypertension. *Anesthesiology*, 33:214, 1970.

Holroyd, S.V. *Clinical Pharmacology in Dental Practice.* C.V. Mosby Co., St. Louis, 1974.

Holvey, D.N. *The Merck Manual*, Ed. 12. Merck, Sharp and Dohme Research Laboratories, Rahway, N.J., 1972.

Hooley, J.R. *Hospital Dentistry.* Lea and Febiger, Philadelphia, 1970.

Howe, G.L., Whitehead, F.I. *Local Anaesthesia in Dentistry.* Williams & Wilkins, Baltimore, 1972.

Hurst, J.W. *The Heart, Arteries and Veins*, Ed. 3. McGraw-Hill Book Co., New York, 1974.

Irby, W.B., Baldwin, K.H. *Emergencies and Urgent Complications in Dentistry.* C.V. Mosby Co., St. Louis, 1965.

Kaplan, E., et. al. Prevention of bacterial endocarditis. *Circulation*, 56:139A, 1977.

Kerr, D.A., Ash, M.M., Jr., Millard, H.D. *Oral Diagnosis*, Ed. 2. C.V. Mosby Co., St. Louis, 1965.

Kimming, J., Jänner, M., Goldsmidt, H. *Corol Atlas of Dermatology.* W.B. Saunders Co., Philadelphia, 1966.

Kirkendall, W.H., Burton, A.C., Epstein, F.H. Recommendation for human blood pressure determination by sphygmomanometer. *Circulation*, 36:980, 1967.

Klostermann, G.F., Südhof, H., Tischendorf, W. *Color Atlas of External Manifestations of Diseases.* McGraw-Hill Book Co., New York, 1964.

Kornel, L., Riddle, M., Schwartz, T.B. The management of hypertension associated with disorders of function of the endocrine glands ("endocrine hypertension"). *Med. Clin. North Am.*, 55:23, 1971.

Krupp, M.A., Chatton, M.J. *Current Diagnosis and Treatment.* Lange Medical Publications, Los Altos, Calif., 1972.

Langley, L.L. *Dynamic Anatomy and Physiology.* McGraw-Hill Book Co. New York, 1974.

Laskin, D.M. *Management of Oral Emergencies.* Charles C Thomas, Springfield, Ill., 1964.

Leake, D., Deykin, D. The diagnosis and treatment of bleeding tendencies. *Oral Surg.*, 32:582, 1971.

Leavell, H.R., Clark, E.G. *Preventive Medicine for the Doctor in his Community*, Ed. 3. McGraw-Hill Book Co., New York, 1965.

Little, J.W. Management of the hypertensive patient in dental practice. *J. Oral Med.*, 29:13, 1974.

MacBryde, C.M., Blacklow, R.S. *Signs and Symptoms: Applied Pathologic Physiology and Clinical Interpretation*, Ed. 5. J.B. Lippincott Co., Philadelphia, 1970.

MacMahon, B., Pugh, T.F. *Epidemiology, Principle and Method.* Little Brown & Co., Boston, 1970.

Malamed, S.F., Sheppard, G.A. *Handbook of Medical Emergencies in the Dental Office.* C.V. Mosby Co., St. Louis, 1978.

Martin, E.W. *Hazards of Medication. A Manual on Drug Interactions, Incompatibilities, Contraindications, and Adverse Effects.* J.B. Lippincott Co., Philadelphia, 1971.

Master, A.M., Lasser, R.P. Blood Pressure Elevation in The Elderly Hypertensive. Recent Advances. Lea and Febiger, Philadelphia, 1961.

Mazzeo, V.A. Physical examination of the head and neck. *J. Oral Med.* (Suppl.) Dec., 1972.

McCarthy, F.M. *Emergencies in Dental Practice, Prevention and Treatment*, Ed. 2. W.B. Saunders Co., Philadelphia, 1972.

McCarthy, F.M. *Emergencies in Dental Practice.* W.B. Saunders Co., Philadelphia, 1967.

Merchant, H.W. Clubbed fingers: indicators of serious disease. *J. Am. Dent. Assoc.*, 96:96, 1978.

Mitchell, D. *Oral Diagnosis/Oral Medicine.* Lea and Febiger, Philadelphia, 1971.

Monheim, L.M. *Local Anesthesia and Pain Control in Dental Practice.* C.V. Mosby Co., St. Louis, 1965.

Moschella, S.L., Pillsbury, D.M., Hurley, H.J. *Dermatology.* W.B. Saunders Co., Philadelphia, 1975.

Odom, J.G., DePaola, D.P., Robbins, A.E. Clinical nutritional education for dental students: a conjoint approach. *J. Am. Diet Assoc.*, 72:56, 1978.

Orkin, L.R. *Management of the Patient in Shock.* F.A. Davis Co., Philadelphia, 1965.

Pearson, R.E. *Anxiety in the Dental Office, Conscious Sedation in Dental Practice.* C.V. Mosby Co., St. Louis, 1974.

Prys-Roberts, C., Meloche, R., Foex, P. Studies of anesthesia in relation to hypertension. I. Cardiovascular response of treated and untreated patient. *Br. J. Anaesth.,* 43:122, 1971.

Ravel, R. *Clinical Laboratory Medicine,* Ed. 2. Year Book Medical Publishers, Chicago, 1973.

Samman, P.D. *The Nails in Disease,* Ed. 2. Charles C Thomas, Publisher, Springfield, Ill., 1972.

Sauer, G.C. *Manual of Skin Diseases,* Ed. 3. J. B. Lippincott Co., Philadelphia, 1973.

Schneewind, J. *Medical and Surgical Emergencies.* Year Book Medical Publishers, Chicago, 1970.

Scopp, I.W. *Oral Medicine,* Ed. 2. C.V. Mosby Co., St. Louis, 1973.

Shafer, W.G., Hine, M.K., Levy, B.M. *A Textbook of Oral Pathology,* Ed. 3. W.B. Saunders Co., Philadelphia, 1974.

Stephenson, H.E. *Cardiac Arrest and Resuscitation,* Ed. 4. C.V. Mosby Co., St. Louis, 1974.

Vernale, C.A. Cardiovascular response to local dental anesthesia with epinephrine in normotensive and hypertensive subjects. *J. Am. Dent. Soc. Anesthesiol.,* 9:133, 1962.

White, R.D. Emergencies in the dental office. *Tex. Dent. J.,* March 20, 1976.

Wilkens, E.M. *Clinical Practice of the Dental Hygienist,* Ed. 3. Lea and Febiger, Philadelphia, 1975.

Wintrobe, M.M. *Clinical Hematology,* Ed. 7. Lea and Febiger, Philadelphia, 1974.

Wintrobe, M.M. et al. *Harrison's Principles of Internal Medicine,* Ed. 7. McGraw-Hill Book Co., New York, 1974.

Wood, P. *Diseases of the Heart and Circulation.* J.B. Lippincott Co., Philadelphia, 1956.

Wood, N.K., Goaz, P.W. *Differential Diagnosis of Oral Lesions. C.V. Mosby Co., St. Louis, 1975.*

Zegarelli, E., Kutscher, A., Hyman, G. *Diagnosis of Diseases of the Mouth and Jaws.* Lea and Febiger, Philadelphia, 1969.

Zinner, S.H., Levy, P.S., Kass, E.H. Familial aggregation of blood pressure in childhood. *N. Engl. J. Med.,* 284:401, 1971.

Additional References

Emergency Care and Transportation of the Sick and Injured. American Academy of Orthopedic Surgeons. Committee on Injuries. G. Banta Co., Menasha, Wis., 1971.

The Third National Cancer Survey; advanced three year report: 1969–1971. National Cancer Institute, Biometry Branch, 1974. DHEW Publication no. (NIH) 74-637, Bethesda, Md.

Standards for Cardiopulmonary Resuscitation (CPR) and Emergency Cardiac Care (ECC). American Heart Association, 1974.

Office Anesthesia Emergency Self-Evaluation Manual. American Society for Oral Surgeons. January, 1971.

Accepted Dental Therapeutics. American Dental Association, Chicago, 1978.

The Merck Manual. Merck and Company, Inc. Rahway, N. J., 1950.

AMA Drug Evaluations. Publishing Sciences Group, Inc., Acton, Mass., 1973.

Dentist responsible for blood pressure screening. *N. Y. State Dent. J.,* 40:430, 1974.

Kiss, F. Tajanatomia. VI Javitott Kiadas. Medicina Konyvkiado, Budapest, 1961.

Index

187